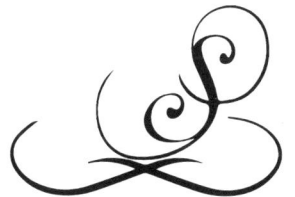

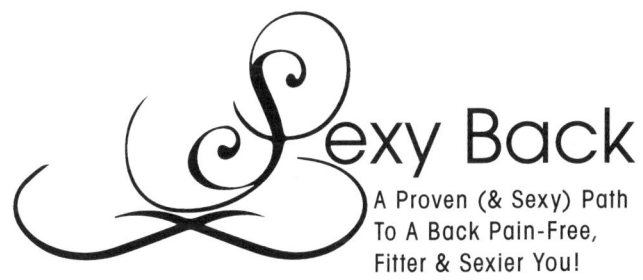

Sexy Back

A Proven (& Sexy) Path
To A Back Pain-Free,
Fitter & Sexier You!

DR. MICHEL RICE

BETTER CALL DOC INC. & SEXY BACK DISCLAIMER

The information provided in Sexy Back by Dr. Michel Rice is designed to provide helpful information on the subjects discussed. Sexy Back is not meant to be used, nor should it be used, to diagnose or treat any medical condition. For diagnosis or treatment of any medical problem, please consult with your family physician. The publisher, Better Call Doc Inc. in association with the printing publisher, Book Baby Inc. and author, Dr. Michel Rice are not responsible for any specific health needs that may require medical supervision and are not liable for any damages or negative consequences from any treatment, action, application or preparation, to any person reading or following the information in this book. Reference citations in the book are provided for informational purposes only and do not constitute endorsement of any websites or other sources.

www.sexybackdoctor.com | info@sexybackdoctor.com

ISBN 978-0-9938394-3-6

Printed in the USA

To my mother Jeannine,
Queen of family love

To my late father George,
Former King of exemplary fatherhood and all things mechanical

To my son Chris,
Master of my life and the FWB relationship

To Louise,
Mistress of my heart & my bedroom

And to my brothers, Rock, Daniel (late 2015) & Pierre
Devout hunters, fishermen, sportsmen & family men

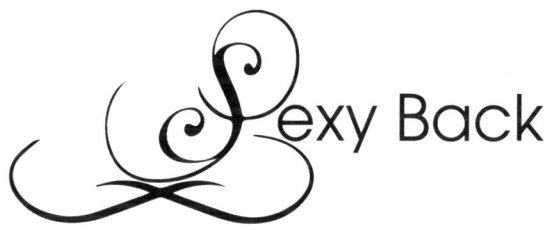

CONTENTS

PREFACE

MY OPENING MONOLOGUE

WELCOME TO SEXY BACK
FEEL SEXY, LOOK SEXY, MOVE WITH SEX APPEAL!
I KNOW YOU WANT TO!

People don't want to exercise to improve their overall health; they're not driven by vital signs or blood chemistry profile. Well, not unless they're under the gun by their health provider.

People are people. For most of us, we exercise to feel sexy, look sexy, and exude sex appeal when we move. We want to look good in clothes. We want our selfies to be hot shots and we feel great for the rest of the day when someone comments on how great we look.

Feel sexy, look sexy, move with sex appeal! Can that explain the billions spent worldwide on plastic surgeries, fantasy web sex sites, fitness businesses, fitness gear, and sexy lingerie? Ya think?

I was motivated years ago to write Sexy Back because it was evident that once a back patient is cured of their pain, what they really want is to feel sexy again. Sex and sexiness are important to patients. So the idea of connecting something more desirable—sex—to exercising for back pain was a good one.

This connection between sex and backs came to me after many female patients explained that their back pain went away when they had good, regular, hot sex.

So that's when the research began. My analytical eye went to work examining the bad asses and the perfect asses in my practice. I was determined to find a way to transform the disabled, sexless lower back into a strong pain-free one using sex as the medicine.

Not too long after the research started came the birth of the Sexy Back club. Then, after completing the manuscript, I shopped it around and was turned off by the attitude and self-serving financial structure of the publishing business. So I held off with the shopping around and I'm glad I did.

IT'S A BOOK…IT'S A CLUB…IT'S A SEX BOOK CLUB!

Sexy Back is a book, not a wellness pamphlet. It's also not a program that you can learn using a short YouTube video. It's a book with a bonus—a prescription (last page of the book) for you to have sex to help you be on your way to fixing your bad back.

The prescription can be used to sway your partner into having back-fixing sex or, even better, help you find a sexy suffering back for you to help fix using the prescription as the ice breaker. So read the book for your pain or read it to learn how to help someone with chronic and crippling back pain. It's a club, remember?

Keep in mind that Sexy Back is also written for you as a solo participant in the program. The 'sexercises' in Sexy III are designed for those who prefer to go solo but use my therapeutic concepts to fix their chronic back pain.

1-2-3-4 THEN TIME TO GET DOWN ON THE FLOOR!

Four facts I want you to know about Sexy Back:

1) You don't need to have sex to fix your back! Although the program gets intimate with sexing and involves a sexy tone throughout the book, you will learn all there is to understanding your back, improving your posture, and learning the secrets to looking twenty pounds lighter and look ten years younger by improving your back condition far beyond your expectations.

2) Sexy Back has all the makings of an educational (well, let's call it medical-entertainment) self-help book. It covers all the necessary subjects to be a complete medical self-help book: anatomy, physiology, pathology, therapy, sex-positionology (I just made that up), sex performance examination and diagnosis, and let's not forget that final exam to test (and certify) your knowledge and new skills! Sexy Back is your go-to source to learn how your spine works, why you have chronic back pain, and how to prevent, control, or fix it. You will benefit tremendously from its power in information.

As a matter of fact, I was careful when writing Sexy Back IV to make sure everyone would be happy—you as a reader and consumer and the medics out there who may want to place judgment upon Sexy Back. To make sure it was complete, I've dissected the content of our past number one bestsellers and cross-referenced my content with these bad back books. Then, I added my work, my theories, my recommendations, my therapies, and added a touch of my Dr. Ricesisms (my own invented words) to make it fun, funny, and memorable for you. I've pretty much reworded and re-explained all the complicated spine stuff with a new and improved way to understand backology— Rice-jargon that you can relate to, remember better, visualize, and enjoy sharing with others.

On top of the standard back book content, I have shared with you my own theories, creations and concepts. These concepts are Millennial-relevant. Medical causes of back pain have spread like the plague among today's millennial generation as much as their predecessors. Sexy Back wouldn't be 'my' book unless I had come up with my own theories and therapies! Otherwise, it would just be a jamboree of other people's work put together in these pages, which is how most self-help books are written. Why bother with that?

No other book in the world shows you how sex can be used as the medicine to fix back pain. Many, mind you, have written a few pages that will teach you how to have sex when your back is crooked and out-of-whack (that's Chapter 13 in my book, entitled Love Hurts)…but to use sex as the therapy of choice? Nope! This is it and it's called Sexy Back!

3) Sexy Back is a program, which means it will take some time to read and practice Sexy Back. Don't be in a rush and don't get your panties in a bunch while doing so. Be patient with your Sexy Back and be patient with the program. It may take some time to learn the sexercises that you first have to learn in Sexy Back. After that, you'll need to spend time learning the program's methodology and guidelines that are to be applied in order to make sex a back-healing experience.

4) Sexy Back is a social media club. It continues to evolve as time goes by. I can attest to that given that I've seen it grow, mature, evolve, and expand in the past 15 years, thanks to your feedback, suffering patient anecdotes, case studies, drunken Sex test trials out in the field (bars, mainly) and even a recent pseudo experiment using my own medical school classmates. It's also evolved thanks to my contributing health professional colleagues' sexperimenting input.

The Sexy Back club starts with the book and then will take you beyond into a higher level of intellectual and physical development through blogging, podcasting, YouTubing, Twittering, guest lecturing, and Instagramming. Bring it on Ms. Social Media! What I'm also really hoping for, deep down, is for a new type of connection to occur between people. Social network connections will occur between groups of people with back pain who don't have partners to help them fix it. And that would be the other group of people—the selfless healers ready to help fix broken back bones once they get with the Sexy Back program. How did you two meet again? Imagine using your medical health records as a means to find a loving partner. Is this a

HIPAA (Health Information Portability and Accountability Act) nightmare or what? Not if you consented!

Because you're now part of the club, I welcome your participation with the help of our social connections...so connect, become a part of our Sexy Back medical community and have some fun will ya?

THE ALTERNATE TITLE CIRCA HBO'S SEX & THE CITY

I started writing Sexy Back in '98. My son was 14 then; he's now 33. I had been practicing for 13 years and have since retired from practice and moved onto a continuing education journey while at the same time conducting medical research trials in the fields of home care medical equipment and traumatic neck injuries resulting from vehicle accidents.

HBO's Sex & the City was a hot television program in '98. Back then, Cosmo girls wanted to be Carrie Bradshaw's best friend and city cowboys wanted to attract those Cosmo girls like Mr. Big did. One day, my witty writer friend, Sheila Muddrick, came up with a great title for the book. At the time, she was a die-hard fan of the show—martini parties with her gay boyfriends every Friday night. Sheila thought I should call the book Sex & the Single Spine Brilliant! It was perfect! The title met with the manuscript's premise: It's about sex, spines, & finding a partner to help fix your single spine! It was sexy and sweet!

So Sex & the Single Spine will remain the alternate title for Sexy Back. After all, it describes the truth behind why most of us would read the book in the first place.

It took me a few years to finish writing the book and it took me even longer to feel comfortable releasing it. Sexy Back deserved more than what Canadian publishers had to offer for first-time authors and I remain, still, protective of it. I wanted better for Sexy back. The book isn't about me nor is it a cry for literary fame (does that even exist in the medical world?). Sexy Back is about you! Sexy Back was written for you, and even by you through shared patient experiences. I was not convinced the time was right to publish it—until now.

THE SEXY BACK PROGRAM AND FITNESS TRAINER CONNECTION

When practicing in Toronto, I was one of the first doctors who pioneered the fitness boutique (hate that word)—a personalized fitness clinic operation that gave you a trainer every time you worked out (love that concept). What? Where are the showers? What do you mean you give me a trainer every time I exercise? I'm allowed to workout in my jeans? A doctor monitors and designs my therapy and recreational exercise program too? Come on, what's it going to cost me?

Now, I can expand on this popular concept by adding the book's program as a specialty certification program for personal fitness trainers. That's what I'm working on now! Class of 2018 graduates will be to sextrain you! The Sexy Back fitness sexperts will guide you through your transformation— new sexy postures for improved back function and sex appeal, new ways to move during all your activities outside the gym, new ways to perform regular exercises you're familiar with, sexercise additions involving osteyoga (yoga for your bones) and core and strength workouts. Their Sexy Back certification makes them authorities on first examining you to help identify your particular physical problem that connects to your back pain. They will then use their specialized sexpertise to help you get to a new level of sexy and fitness you never thought you could attain—improved back function, pain control, sexual performance and a new sexy you. Having a trainer with a specialty in sexercise is going to make you above all other trainer programs—it's a sexy social status.

It all comes down to this…feel sexy, look sexy, and move with sex-appeal! With the advent of social media and e-medicine, the Sexy Back specialty trainer certification program will allow me to reach you, to get closer to you, to understand your individual needs and desires, and to make sure that you get what you want out of the program through me directly or my sexician certified team in a club near you.

WWW.SEXYBACK.CLUB—NOT NET AND NOT COM

The publication process is tightly connected to you via social media networks. The time to release Sexy Back is now! What I am most excited about is how the book can become a part of you via print copies, audio, electronic transcriptions, and as mentioned above, how you can get involved with the club via social outlets. You can speak about it and be heard worldwide. You can advertise for help, asking for a partner to fix your chronic back pain and someone will come knocking on your iPhone to help. You can advertise yourself as being the best healer in town and just maybe the patient of your dreams may want your personal sexician services, until death do you part? Imagine that! Posting, uploading, downloading, and commenting can be as big as the book itself. That's what I want for Sexy Back. It will be a growing community of praises—with rants and raves also welcomed. It can be your source to connect and your source to get answers. Welcome to the Sexy Back club. Read on…

1

WHAT THE WORLD NEEDS NOW IS LOVE... & LESS BACK PAIN

Pretty much everything can be hard or soft wired to sex! Advertising, entertainment, fashion, sports and food all direct us down the slippery slope to getting sex, having sex and enjoying sex.

So why do people have less and less sex?

There are a handful of things that prevent sex, like sexual dysfunction, psychological problems and faulty plumbing, but in my practice the number one thing that leads to no sex is back pain.

Huh? Who would have thought...back pain leads to no sex! If I were to ask you which came first, back pain or no sex, the answer gets complicated. Back pain kills sex but... fancy drum roll...sex prevents back pain. There is a clinical connection between your sex life (or lack thereof) and your back pain.

It is my plan to show you that sex is a remedy for back pain and that sex is the best exercise to prevent back pain. For once the cure is much better than the disease—and, might I add, considerably more fun. Of course, this also means that the lack of sex in your life could have been the cause of your back pain this whole time! Have you needlessly sacrificed your most enjoyable activity for no reason other than the myth that "a bad back means bad sex"?

The sexual revolution began decades ago, so for all you medical martyrs, I apologize for creating this program thirty years too late. From now on things will be different. Your new philosophy will be "Honey, my back is killing me. Let's sexercise it away." These are the Doctor's orders!

FROM LAID UP TO GETTING LAID

So what am I pushing? How to use sex to cure your bad back? Or how to have sex with your bad back? The answer is both. I'm going to give you a lot of the "sex-as-therapy-for-your-chronic-low-back-pain" advice, with a small dose of "how-to-take-pleasure-in-sex-when-your-back-feels-like-it-a-steak-knife-running-though-it" advice.

So is the subject mainly about sex? Yes! All things lead to sex. Including curing back pain. Having sex during an acute back pain episode requires a basic understanding of which positions are safe, which are bad and which are just too hot for you. I will teach you to be naughty in bed without being nasty to your back.

Still skeptical? Well, let me give you all the advance warning I can. This is a book about the human body, its need for pleasure and its intolerance for pain. It is both graphic and comforting. We all know sex is hard to avoid in our society. So is back pain. I intend to give you graphic sexual advice to heat up your sex life and at the same time fix your chronic back pain. I'm going to give you both hot, sexy advice and practical, precise, clinical advice. What you do with it is up to you.

2

THE SISY SQUAT
SEX TEST

In my practice I have seen thousands of patients with varying degrees of flexibility, fitness and pain. In the process I have developed a simple test to determine the integrity of the human torso. Actually, it's better than that. It can tell if you have a strong enough back to be a titillating sexual partner. It can also tell you if someone else has a strong enough back to be an optimum sexual partner for you. Aside from the fact that my test can help millions of people in the age-old search for good old sex, passing my little test is everyone's goal. I call this test The Sisy Squat Sex Test.

Anyone who has worked out in a weight room knows the maneuver called the sissy squat, whereby, with a weight plate held to your chest, you bend your knees while rising up on your toes, and slowly lower yourself toward the floor until your buttocks almost touch your heels. Then straighten your legs and repeat. I have created a version of this maneuver that tests the characteristics necessary in the making of a strong and pain-free spine that I call "The Sisy Squat Sex Test". The word "Sisy" is not taken from the word sissy squat. It is derived from Sisyphus, the Greek King of Corinth—more about him in a minute. The Sisy Squat Sex Test can be used as a self-examination tool (if you're brave enough to self-test), secondly, as a conversation piece (a slick little ice-breaker), or thirdly, to determine if a potential partner is worthy of an invitation back to your place (a deal breaker). Just drop a hanky (i.e., ask them to do The Sex Test) and see how they perform. Your sexy specimens will never know about your wicked intentions unless you tell them.

Why do we like self-examination tests? Why do we get tempted to test ourselves so easily? Every magazine has a variation on the Cosmo Quiz, and everyone I know completes them. Yet, rarely does anyone do anything to take the next step toward self-improvement. Furthermore, I have not known anyone to actually take the time to complete a "How Bad is Your Back?" self-test questionnaire, let alone follow through with its recommendations. Why would they? How many people do you know who would be motivated to make sure their "L5-S1 complex was mechanically intact without particular dysfunctions or myofascial strain"? I think we both know that answer.

In spite of our inherent reluctance to use the advice of the self-help questionnaire, we are still very curious about self-help scores. Finding out if you're a speed freak, cliff-walker, drifter, worrywart, or control freak is only useful if it puts you at ease to know that you're just like everyone else! We all want to know if we "fit in."

The other day, my son's friend Omar asked me to take Maxim Magazine's S.A.T. (Sexual Aptitude Test), designed to determine if you know the "ins and outs" of sex. He handed me a pencil, the magazine, and a folded piece of paper with his own answers on the other side. For a moment I panicked. What if I wasn't up to snuff? What if he actually scored higher than me? What would my son think of his dad, author of Sexy Back? Luckily, Omar muttered a dare that brought me to my senses.

His score? Between 1,080 and 1,270, which meant, according to Maxim, he had "clearly had some direct experience with sex, or he could afford explicit magazines and internet clubs." My score? On the cusp of the highest possible score: 1,480. Thank goodness! I was relieved until I read Maxim's comment: "What's it like to be me? A big f*@#- ing liar? What's the real score, chump?" I went from a high-scoring stud to a dud in a millisecond, which brings us to the other major problem with self-tests (particularly ones found in men's glossies): most self-tests mean nothing. Most self-tests prove nothing.

My test, on the other hand, is not useless. The Sisy Squat Sex Test works and in a minute I'll show you how to do it, and soon you too will victimize many innocent people by getting them to unknowingly reveal how their bedroom performance rates. Why is my test not useless? It is both a test and an exam! It is pass or fail and there is no possibility of cheating. In the battle of the sexes it is the perfect measure of whether or not the duel of love is worth the bother.

Here are my top five reasons why my sex test is a valuable clinical commodity for both your social life and your sex life:

Time Management: Who's got time to waste when the target is standing two feet away and it's five minutes to last call? Egad...and you're still not sure?

Lie Detector Test: The Sisy Squat Sex Test is an excellent yet unobtrusive way to see if the braggart is all he claims to be.

Vanity and Self Discoveries: Performing The Sisy Squat Sex Test in the privacy of your bedroom provides a terrific indicator to measure the successes of your Sexy Back program. The Sisy Squat Sex Test is a before, during, and after success-measuring tool.

Group Therapy: Share your Sisy Squat Sex Test magic trick with your friends. I guarantee it will keep them talking and, for more than a few of them, crying.

Scare Tactics: Use the Sex Test to scare them off! Dare any potential lover or pest to try it. It'll weed out the weenies. But be careful, you might start reconsidering the pests if they pass the test with flying colors.

One more bit of exposition before we get to the nitty-gritty of The Sisy Squat Sex Test:

YOU DON'T KNOW SQUAT: A BEDTIME STORY BY UNCLE MICHEL

Once upon a time, there lived a King of Corinth called Sisyphus (Sis-i-fus), who was known to be the most cunning, sly, and sneaky little bastard on earth (who said this was a children's bedtime story?). When Hades, the god of the underworld, finally had it with the king's wicked ways, he came personally to claim Sisyphus for the kingdom of the dead. Expecting Sisyphus to weasel out—or at least put up a struggle—Hades brought along a pair of handcuffs, a novelty for those times. Sisyphus cunningly expressed an interest in the "never seen before" handcuffs. His interest was so great that Hades was persuaded by Sisyphus to try them out on himself! In an instant Hades was handcuffed, at Sisy's mercy and hidden away. For years, as the god of the underworld was kept from hell, nobody on earth could die. In battle after battle soldiers were knifed, stabbed, choked and ripped apart, but still made it to back to camp in time for a dry bun and a tin cup of beans and wieners.

Years later Hades was released and Sisyphus was once again ordered to report to the underworld for his eternal assignment. Our shifty king made some quick arrangements and ordered his dutiful wife not to bury his body when he died. So Sisyphus remained unburied and filed an appeal with Persephone, Queen of the Dead. Luckily for Sisyphus, Persephone sided with his complaint that his unburied corpse needed a more formal, ceremonial funeral. Not surprisingly, Sisyphus did everything but make arrangements for his own funeral. But his time came again and Hades finally dragged him down to the underworld to receive a final sentence for all his indiscretions.

For having committed the worst of crimes, a crime against the gods, Hades decided to return Sisyphus back to earth for a lifetime of hard labor? His punishment? Sisyphus had to roll the biggest of boulders to the top of a steep hill, only to have the boulder roll back down for him to do all over again. Eternally. No labor union, no ergo knee pads, no family benefit plan, and no coffee break either! The end. (Sort of).

THE SISY SQUAT SEX TEST

Imagine the position you would take in order to push a heavy boulder up a hill. In bodybuilder culture the sissy squat is indeed as grueling as pushing a boulder the size of a city bus tire up a hill. Most bodybuilders perform the sissy squat in sets and reps. The Sisy Squat Sex Test, as it applies to our sneaky secret test that rates sexual performance, is a modified version of the bodybuilders' sissy squat. I've taken the boulder away and made Sisyphus bend down a little more than he had to in order to push the rock up the hill. Like the King pushing the boulder, the crouch position is the finish point of the test. If you can get down there, you pass. How you get there, however, is another story.

You have your choice of three variations. Option one: take your shoes off and place them on the floor in front of you with the toe part of your shoe facing your own toes. Stand on the toe part of your shoe and keep your heels on the floor. Option two: stand facing a wall, feet shoulder width apart and toes one inch from the wall. Option three is the more engaging option: have someone stand in front of your with toe-to-toe contact. The toe-to-toe position is more difficult to execute because it limits your forward swing.

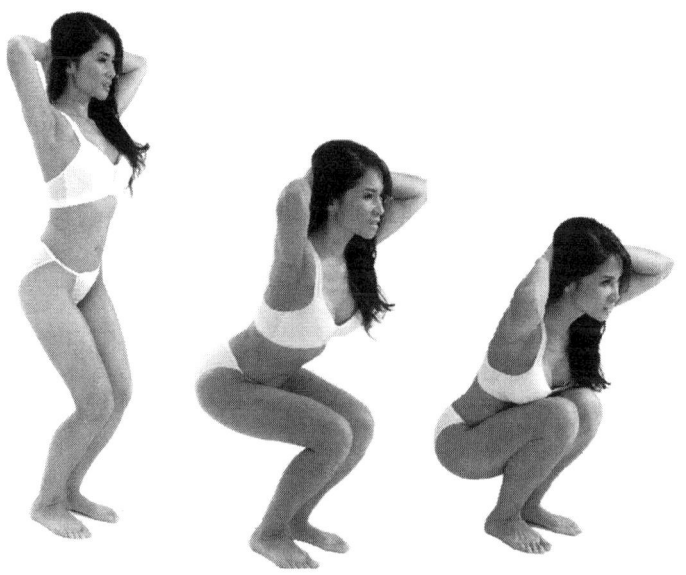

Place your hands behind your head like you're going to be arrested. Although three lower limb positions have been described here, the standard position is the toe-to-toe contact with the examiner and your hands behind your head. This is the one I use as my base to see if you pass or not. All other variations are to avoid embarrassment and account for sobriety.

THE ACTION

Toes well-positioned, feet shoulder-width apart, heels on the floor the entire time, with eyes facing forward, start squatting your way down, slowly and steadily. Your end-point should be ass almost to the floor, chest behind (not above or in front of) your knees, and eyes—well, let's just say they should be positioned right at the…er…finish line. Remember that your heels must stay on the floor the entire time. Any other way would be cheating. Performing this maneuver without falling backwards is the mark of a passed test. Coming back up is not part of The Sisy Squat Sex Test.

This maneuver is complex when dissected with a clinical eye. The Sisy Squat Sex Test leaves no room for the disadvantaged spine—disadvantaged from the loss of agility, the weakening of abdominals, and the lessening of ass curves (concepts I will be explaining in depth in the pages to come and which you will need to understand if you want to fix your chronic back problem with sex). The Sisy Squat Sex Test is the ultimate indicator of a working spine. You have already learned that it has many uses, be it the pick-up ticket, sex therapist, marriage counselor, or self-improvement indicator. It is the guide that will tell you if you're better in bed than you think you are or if your marriage can be saved with this program's lovemaking prescription. If you can pass The Sisy Squat Sex Test, there is nothing you can't do.

What if your partner did not pass the test? Fear not. You will soon know what to do with your sex partner. I'm going to teach you how to fix their backs using sex and make big improvements to your own!

3

WHAT'S THAT BEHIND MY BACK?

Let's face it…backs are boring! For most of us it takes a stabbing pain to make us even think about our backs. Sadly, by this time, life will have taken a turn for the worse. First, you limit activity. Then, you limit sex. You can't sleep comfortably. You take pills. Pills curb your sex drive. Now you avoid sex altogether. It's a fast ride to the bottom of the hill. Love dries up. Sleep disappears. Depression sets in. Your gut starts to bulge. Your only friends live at addresses that begin with www.

Some people think of their back as an annoying parasite, quietly living inside them with the occasional unexpected flare-up. A lot of people even think it looks like a parasitic bug. Looking at a picture of an upside-down spine on my desk, one patient actually asked me what kind of bug it was. Imagine that! He was in a back clinic with back pain talking to a back doctor about his back and thought the doctor had bug pictures on his desk!

People talk about their back like it's not part of their being: "How was your holiday?" "Fine thanks!" "And how was your back?" "Back was fine, too!" Some people talk as if their back is a temperamental child: "How's the back doing, Flo?" "Not too bad, Clint. It's been pretty good lately. Hasn't acted up for some time now. Lucky, I guess? Knock on wood." Flo considers herself very lucky, as if there is nothing she can do about her unpredictable, uncontrollable back tantrums.

WHEN IT COMES TO YOUR BACK, IT'S OUT-OF-SIGHT, OUT-OF-MIND.

Maybe we would pay more attention to our backs if the spine were like a parasitic bug or at least a slimy, gooey textured organ that spits out blood in gushing pulses when we "throw our backs out"? Have I piqued your interest? Any shivers running down your spine now?

For better or for worse, our fears are not triggered by the potential for back pain. It doesn't scare us like internal bleeding, intestinal blockages, brain aneurysms, kidney stones, heart attacks, breast cancer, or third degree burns do. How sympathetic was your boss the last time your back went out? For most of us the spine is merely the centerpiece of the stick man. Nothing more. Yet a back injury can stop you dead in your tracks. The late Christopher Reeve has drawn attention to the risks but still, how many of you are really scared that a terrible, debilitating back injury could happen to you? No movement, no voluntary muscle action, no respirator, no breath.

NO BREATH, NO LIFE!

Yet, people are bored by backs. And back books are no help. Browsing through my local bookstore I see that back books are big business. More than one has a blurb that brags, "Over 1,000,000 copies in print." Based on my experience, I think the blurb should read, "More than 1,000,000 copies in print, less than 100,000 sold, less than 10,000 read cover-to-cover, less than 1,000 tried the program, and less than 100 persisted longer than 10 days." No one reads back books because back books are dull. Let's face it: When it comes to your back, it's out-of-sight, out-of-mind.

Big back books, small back books, hardback and paperback. I've read them all. I long to answer questions like "Why do even the worst of back pain sufferers still find backs boring?" Not enough pictures? Too much technical jargon? Exercises too difficult to follow? Too much information to remember? Format too technical? Advice not realistic? The answer definitely lies in a combination of many factors.

Ever skim through a medical journal? It becomes apparent why back books are so boring when you examine the medical peer review journals for those physicians who write back books in the first place. Reading the Parkhurst Exchange Medical Journal, it becomes clear that one of the tactical tricks of the Journal editors is to strategically place comic strips every few pages. The last issue I read had 24 cartoons in a 130-page spread, to be exact! When the subject involves backs, even physician's journals need entertainment to keep our attention.

So what makes Sexy Back so different from all the other back books? For one thing, sex enters a man's thought process approximately once every 20 minutes. If a man sleeps eight hours a night, it means that I have at least 48 invitations a day to remind a guy, with or without pain, to read Sexy Back for his back's sake. "Nice legs…smells good…need sex… back hurts…must read Sexy Back" It's a fairly straightforward thought process. With Sexy Back, the mechanics connecting sex thoughts with back thoughts become as simple a process as the knee-jerk reflex—hand in fire…finger hot…finger very hot…finger burning…pull back…save finger! Sex is a reflex. It is a need that requires no thought. That is why it was easy to recognize, create, and implement the concept that such a simple need (sex) could be used to solve a complex problem (back pain). Luckily, the clinical, mechanical, and physiological basis behind Sexy Back's sex-back pain connection generously backs up the fact that sex is actually very good for back pain. And since I have approximately 1,440 monthly invitations to activate a man's cerebral and limbic sex/back neuron connections, imagine my odds for women!

Sexy Back is not a gimmick wish book, nor is it a medical school textbook, nor is it a Yin-Yang tea bag remedy recipe, nor is it an "all talk—no action" back care reference text. Sexy Back is a hands-on list of activities for better back health, for pain-free sex and for sex to be pain-free.

You've already been served a tasty appetizer called The Sisy Squat Sex Test—a test that can secretly help you determine if your potential playmate is lousy in bed, or badly in need of a crash course on back-fixing intercourse. Next is my movable feast, a description of the principles needed to understand why my sexercise program works. These are teaser chapters that explain how important sex HELP YOU KISS YOUR SORE BACK GOODBYE is for your low back pain without giving you the juicy 'how to' just yet. These principles are the succulent hors d'oeuvres of your five-course meal.

Next on the menu is the meaty course of the book: The Wham Bam Program. Wham Bam has two sections. The first part covers the sexercises: the juiciest hanky-panky movements that will help you kiss your sore back goodbye as you kiss your newfound sex appeal hello. The next part is practical, the hands-on turn-on that will forever change your views about exercise and make you a firm believer that practice makes perfect.

For those of you who are acutely in pain with a whole bunch of unanswered questions about how to make sex-play safe and enjoyable, I come to your rescue in the "Love Hurts" chapter of Sexy Back. It's your first-aid emergency care that will help keep your lumbar pain away while you passionately play.

For dessert I share with you how to put together your newfound skills and test your newly acquired powers with the 15 most common sexual positions. Are these positions safe for her? Can his back stand the test of time in this position? The program is easy to follow and you will savor each course as you become an expert in the field of sex with low back pain and sex for low back pain. Bon appétit!

Who am I and what qualifies me to write about sex and spines? For one thing, having the same body parts and drive as any healthy Homo sapiens unquestionably gives me an upper hand in writing about the first part of Sexy Back: sex! As far as the spine is concerned, I just so happen to have one of my own. The difference is that unlike most people, I pay attention to it. Is it because I am a doctor? Probably so, but I was paying attention long before I got into a grueling ten years of post-secondary education.

My credibility as an expert in the bondage of back pain and sex is justified by two prerequisites. First, by my patients' shared sexual experiences involving both their spinal malfunction and self-repair techniques. Second, by my fitness bliss, which has had overspill benefits in pointing out the useful and picking out by the handful the back care exercise faddy rubbish that exists out there. I've been practicing what I've been preaching for more than 25 years!

On top of my extensive clinical experiences with bad back attacks, my privileged opportunities in having talked to well over 10,000 patients have given me an entertaining advantage. "Having trouble with traditional positions? Talk to me!" "Feel better after you do what?! Tell me more!" I was quick to realize the natural connection between a patient's freedom from low back pain and sex. After making this connection I proceeded to gather the clinical information needed to back me up and allow me to share my discoveries.

Sexy Back will give you an easy lift to new and improved physical possibilities and a prescription for adventure. For those of you not so fortunate as to have a honey around the house to help with your suffering— a not-by-choice marital status I call the suffering sexless single "spiner"—you will find at the end the world's most valuable ticket to a sure pick-up tactic: a prescription to help you pick out a partner to help you ease your way back to spinal health. Of course, the prescription for copulation was deliberately placed at the back of the book. This ticket to a better and improved sexercise life is to be used only after reading all preceding chapters. Knowing why is just as important as knowing how.

My plan will help you help yourself and help you identify the one who can also help you. Hopefully, you will be one of the lucky ones who will have their prescription filled in no time at all. And if you're on a real lucky streak, your health plan may even cover some of the costs involved. Save that nightcap, cab ride, and back book receipt! Could corporate health benefits get any better? Sure, how about having a Sexy Back seminar with me as presenter. Be prepared to laugh, love and learn!

On the down side if your prospective fantasy nursing applicant turns out to be turned off by your request for a sexy back fixing session, don't worry—just keep reading. If I were attentive enough to come up with the idea that sex will optimize your spinal hygiene, then you can bet that I made sure to cover all possible positions that you just may find yourself in. Sexy Back is not only for the "single and very willing to go shopping;" it's also for the "no-go because I'm a strict solo" or the "abstain is my main game" patron. Sexy Back is guaranteed to cover your ambition to have a healthy spine—with, or without a partner…to bed, or not to bed…with or without sex!

Why Are You Reading this Book? Are you reading because you've had it with your bad back and now is the time to care? Have you experienced any of the following?

- Your back goes out more often than you do (okay, the joke may be as tired as your back is, but the problem is real!);
- You're so hunchbacked you only recognize your friends by the type of shoes they wear;
- You opt out of the Heimlich maneuver because you know those squeezing back thrusts will hurt more than death itself by choking;
- You waste your birthday candle wishes on ridding yourself of back pain;
- You list your back as a dependant on your tax return;
- You sign the back of your driver's license as a "spinal organ" donor for research;
- You can't be bothered to wipe the frozen snot running down your upper lip because blowing your nose just hurts your back too much; or

Are you reading because you want to find out about sex? Sex to fix your back? Sex every day of the week? And last of the Top Ten List? For sex!

HOW WILL YOU KEEP MOTIVATED?

If your spine were a different person living in your body, how would you describe its personality? Irritable? Bitchy? Pain in the butt? Moody? Unpredictable? Stubborn? Temperamental? If your back were a motor vehicle what would it be? Truck? Chip stand? Hearse? These are questions that reflect the real reason why you want your back pain to go away. The funny thing is that when learning the art of taking a medical history this question should always be asked: What is the real reason you want your pain to stop? But the problem is, even if the question is asked, you never know if your doctor is listening.

Can you talk to your doctor?

"Doctor, I'm concerned about the osteophyte growths on the vertebral endplates of my fifth lumbar vertebra!" the patient complains.

"Oh my goodness—so am I. Your radiographs indicate a moderate stage of degenerative disc disease!" the doctor replies.

"Oh great, let's begin therapy right away. I can't imagine what my x-rays would look like if I didn't pursue treatment immediately. Can we arrest the development of more vertebral slipping?"

"Doctor, ever since you showed me the subchondral sclerosis in my low back, I'm having trouble sleeping at night. I'm very worried about this condition progressing into a degenerative arthropathy."

"Oh my goodness—let's get you some atypical anti-depressants. This should help you sleep better, worry less, and, you know, feel better about your life. Your subchondral sclerosis won't bother you a bit after that."

Does your doctor understand that you need to stay awake, sleep around, loosen up and rid yourself of your degenerative 'attitudinopathy'?

Does your doctor listen to you when you talk about your real life? "Doctor, I'm serious. I'm very anxious about this new symptom. I've never felt this before. I think I need to have you perform nerve root provocation tests on my back. When I'm sitting on the john, my right leg goes numb!" as the patient shares her* innermost feelings with the doctor. (*Okay Okay! I know this only happens to guys on the john!)

"Oh my goodness, let's do the Valsalva orthopedic test right away. Heck, while we're at it, let's do all other relevant nerve root provocation tests, too—just to make sure! I sure hope your nerve root isn't involved."

No true patient is concerned about osteophytes, degenerative arthropathy, subchondral sclerosis, Valsalva, nerve root irritation, or body parts called lumbar number five. Nobody cares about the anatomical details of their dysfunctional body parts. The only time it becomes convenient to use the medical jargon is when the boss asks why you took the day off. Patients need life! Doctors need to get involved with the life the patient is trying to keep. That's why people get back treatments, day after day, receiving time-consuming therapy and listening to boring advice on sleeping, sitting, standing, lifting, and paying for it on the way out! I believe this to be the truth and the inner drive behind your present time with Sexy Back. It's really not to make the pain go away—drugs can do that! We persist with treatment programs that promise to make us move with ease and power—to give us freedom to move smoothly and without worry through the adventures of our day-to-day life.

Think about what makes you tick and use it to make you stick with this program. What's it going to take to turn you into a tenacious little eager beaver to fix your bad back? Will you stick to the program for motorcycling? For golfing? For walking and hiking? For your cycling, swimming, or skiing? Chances are it will be for anything that ends with an "ing," so find the thing you like to do, click with it and stick to it. You're doing it for a better quality of life—for freedom of body movement and freedom of live-"ing"!

DOCTORS NEED TO GET INVOLVED WITH THE LIFE THE PATIENT IS TRYING TO KEEP

One more personal and meaningful incentive that may be a positive factor in keeping your eyes (and life) in focus with the Sexy Back program is to keep your sex life ticking. To melt the ice that's been keeping the temperature under the bedspread at forty below for years. To learn how to screen out lousy sex partners. For a few laughs. To be more understanding toward sufferers of low back pain. To have more (and better) sex.

And if sex is not enough to keep you focused, how about fear?

First there was Scream I. Then came the sequels, Scream II and III. And now comes its spin-off: Fear I. The plot of Fear I is simple. It is the very first episode of back pain. Screams, shrieks, and screeches are the main theme till finally a hair-raising Ouch! ends it all. A scary spectacle, but the pain and the plot ended, never to return. But...

Then comes Fear II: The Sequel. The insane pain makes its second coming just when you thought it was safe to go out. The drug overdose you used to kill it in Fear I was not enough! You screamed a lot louder in Fear II (nothing worthy of an Oscar nod, mind you) but then the pain was killed—again.

Unfortunately, you were left with the nagging feeling that maybe this time Mr. Pain might have survived its second killing—again. Was the post-climactic closing of Fear II deliberately arranged to leave a little room for another sequel? Well, you know the answer, only the story line has changed a tad.

The third coming of recurrent back pain is more than a little scary plot laden with the screams of yet another victim crying for help. It's bigger than that now. Can't turn the clock back to the good old days when a little screaming, a little resting, and a little drugging could make the pain go away. This recurrent horror production can best be described as a blend of psychological thriller and sheer horror. Coming to a body near you is the new psychological horror feature: Fear III. "Damn it, here we go again!" You panic—you freeze. This time, you remember how painful it was the last time it visited you. "How much more of this can I take?" The third time pain makes its special appearance you are horrified. You now live in fear! Could you possibly be the big, shiny, screaming star of this picture?

What do you call people who cancel dates because they're afraid their backs will go out? What kind of life do people have when they start avoiding events that require even the dinkiest of physical energy like sitting: sitting on a park bench...sitting at an anniversary dinner party...sitting in an 18-wheeler truck...sitting in a movie theater...sitting for a car ride...or sitting on public transit. Sitting! What do you call those people? I call them backophobics...people who live in fear, controlled by their back pain.

Stories of fear are life's horror films, leaving you forever looking over your shoulder, afraid of the unknown. The fear of an unknown is worse than fear itself. You don't know when the bomb's going to go off—the etiological factor. You don't know what the heck is wrong with you—the diagnosis. You don't understand a word of your condition after it has been explained to you—the complicated report of examination findings. You don't know what position to put yourself in so as not to make it worse—the relieving factor. You don't know what sets off the back attacks—the triggering factor. You can't predict when the attack will recur—the unknown pathophysiological sequelae. You don't know how much more of this you can take—the complete whacko breakdown!

Living in fear is one good reason to seek out help. And the kind of fear you have is a good step toward defining your problem. If fear is the scary monstrosity you've been waiting for before screaming for help, the problem will usually be labeled as chronic in nature. Acute pains will usually tie you down for a short while and force you to take a day off or two. Acute pain's sharp and poignant character, staying with your every move, will create the fright experienced during a fresh back attack. The acute screams are maximal. After a few recurrent episodes or when acute pain turns ugly because it's really overstayed its welcome, then the problem becomes chronic. Pain is chronic when it hangs around longer than three months. Usually, by the time fear has set in, a lot of damage has been done. If brain fear is induced by recurrent episodes of unpredictable back breakdowns, imagine the effect those recurrent physical forces have had on the spine, let alone your brain. It takes a lot of pain to change scary feelings into fearful feelings. It takes a lot of fear to say no to a good movie, a hot date, or happy hour.

So do I think you should use fear to steer yourself to better health? Yes! Am I kidding? I'm afraid not! If fear is why you are here, then take a deep breath, walk toward the light, welcome it, and use it to your advantage. Fear can be a good thing! You can let it be your drive to fix the problem.

Another kind of fear sets in when you look into the mirror and you see the naked truth about yourself. You are wearing a flesh-colored life belt around your waist. But after your second glance you realize it was just one of those mirror tricks. Faster than you can say "holy degenerative disc disease", your inner dialogue speaks out: "Oh! My! Gawd! When did this happen to me?"

An overblown tale of blubber, you may think? Not so. Gaining weight is a mere side effect of living in fear. When activity goes down it takes your spirit down, too. The weight slowly piles on and makes you move a little slower every day. The extra belly flab around your waist begins to change your bra size, your belt size, and your moods. Making matters worse, the extra poundage adds to the physical stresses on your sore back. And the cycle continues: the pain creates more fear...fear sedates all desires for activity...inactivity contributes to more weight gain...and the weight gain creates more back pain. See the pattern? Feel the fear? Pain, fear, inactivity, weight gain, pain, fear, inactivity, weight gain, home alone. Again.

How do you stop the life rings from growing? First, you must find the mental strength within and use it to help develop the spinal strength within.

OLDER AND BETTER

So why are you here? Getting rid of your fear and that paunchy belly are two good reasons to get you back into the life-love swing of things. Here's another: "teeners" are out—"agers" are in! Youth is out and graceful aging is in! Our 21st century earthly population is growing older. In 1996, approximately one in ten was a senior. The United Nation's Department of Economics and Social Affairs predicts that the number of older persons has tripled over the last 50 years; it will move than triple again over the next 50 years. The older population is growing faster than the total population in practically all regions of the world—and the difference in growth rates is increasing. Imagine the competition for handicapped parking spots! We are living in a world of agers, and the agers will go a long way to make sure they ripen as gracefully as possible.

ADD as a last sentence in that paragraph: Thank you Dr. Ho for your innovative senior-care medical product developments—Boom Care is in!!!

Agers rule and elder-conscious businesses are on the bandwagon. Adult-only complexes, retirement homes, nursing home establishments, and senior citizen health care centers are booming. The internal youthful feeling, however, is not as easy to come by. With the advancement of preventive cancer screens, the big ones can be cured, controlled, or at

> TO AGE GRACEFULLY IS TO MOVE ELEGANTLY INTO LIFE'S THIRD TRIMESTER

least held up significantly longer than if left untreated. Then there are these extraordinary, golden ideas such as adult-sized diapers (three pees per pair and you're still dry... imagine that), the coronary bypass and stents, and the omnipotent Viagra, to name a few.

Geriatrics has become a gigantic medicinal and commercial sector. What about the musculo-skeletal (muscles and bone) area of gerontology? The goal of geriatric treatment is one of anti-freezing: keeping things moving, relieving pain and discomfort, preventing deterioration and disability, and improving the quality of life. Without freedom from low back pain and without freedom of movement, you lose a big chunk of your life. True freedom is "never having to feel your back hurt."

For the aged, graceful means supple, flexible, limber, agile, pliable, independent, and active. For me, to age gracefully is to move elegantly into life's third trimester—

a classic reason why you should want to care for your back. For most, however, elegant aging is not on their list of "things to do today to better my health tomorrow." Most people either don't really get it or don't really care.

In the opposite corner, we have the "a penny saved is a penny earned" patron who believes in taking care of things now for a better future—fully functional, runs as good as new, and still has original body parts...it's a classic! Ah! Now there's a reason why you should pay attention now rather than later!

Keep all of your original body parts and run as good as new even when you're not so new anymore.

But there is more to good personal health than good physical health. I believe expressing yourself—expressing your mind and soul—is an important component of good personal health. I believe there are Vows of Self Expression: Do what you want to do. Do what you've gotta do. Come as you like. Say what's on your mind. Do as you feel. Express your true feelings. Express yourself. Be yourself. Do what makes you happiest. Go for it! I know it's not easy to keep these vows with back pain. I ask you to take care of your spine to live life fully. Be "spineful," not spineless.

4

THE KNEE BONE'S CONNECTED TO THE...

The exam at the end of the Gettin' Kissy Kissy Chapter is open book style. Get a feel for the concepts, i.e., the steering wheel controls direction, motor means power, and power means getting from point A to point B in record time. If you understand the concepts, then you will pass—I promise! You don't need Gray's Atlas of Human Anatomy, with its splendid spinal spread amongst its 1,247 vibrant engravings.

On the other hand, do not expect your Flesh 'n Bones instruction manual to be at the least level of difficulty. It would be too easy to point to your ass, low back, and pelvis and just call that the complete guide to spinal anatomy. Our "spineology" lesson, however, will be appropriate and painless.

...THE GREAT CURVE

Let's begin with surface anatomy. Take a rear view of your partner. You are facing the essential body element that keeps your body erect: a big, rigid and fleshy pillar called your spinal column. Six inches above the uppermost portion of your gluteal cleft (the butt crack) there lies the base of your lumbar spine. Pronounced like "lum" as in a stiff piece of lumber, and "bar" as in Stella Artois at happy hour. Lumbar is the name given to the section of your spine that makes up your low back.

There are two more parts to your spine: the cervical spine is the neck part of your spine and the thoracic spine is the thorax part of your spine. From a side view, you should be able to see a dipping lumbar curve that is shaped like a half moon. This curve, called the lordosis, is meant to be! Your lordosis is what gives your ass a nice shape, making it look firm and round, sticking out and ready to lure the wandering eye.

From a posterior view (staring at someone's backside from the back), you will notice the same lumbar dip just above your posterior. Unlike halitosis and hyperhydrosis (stinky breath and sweaty palms), a lordosis is not a bad thing to have. It's the name we have given to your curvy lumbar spine. When each bony soldier is in place, one vertebra on top of the other, the lordotic curve it creates is stable. This mature curve needs minimal muscle activity to hold it together.

If the lordosis curve is not so perfect, it carries a prefix that identifies what exactly went wrong with it. A hyperlordosis means there's too much there, hence, "hyper". A hypolordosis (hype-oh, not hip-o) means there is not enough there. Most of us are hypos. We have evolved into hypos with flat asses. This is the resulting evolutionary development from a long life of ass-sitting activity. The "Flat Ass Syndrome" has become so common that it has very likely made its way into our chromosome genome pool. "Yup! I got my father's eyes and his flat ass, too!"

As we rest on our rears for years, our lordosis slowly disappears. We are chronically sedentary sitting sapiens. We have turned into billions of sitting ducks just waiting for discs to blow over, decay, and progress to degenerative arthropathy (a diseased or impaired joint) faster than a compost heap filled with last week's catch of the day— fish heads and all. If you are a hypolordotic—the majority of us—your bones are perfectly malpositioned to start giving you disc-type pain. Chronic disc irritation will turn around and bite you right in the ass.

If you are hyperlordotic the excess curve may be giving you the nicest looking ass in the neighborhood but the accentuated curve will eventually irritate the apophyseal joints of your lumbar bones. Discs are at the front of the spine and apophyseal joints are at the back of the spine (more about apophyseal joints later). With either "hyper" or "hypo" you cannot win. Damned if you are too much and damned if you aren't enough!

To sum up, if you're a deviant from lordosis, being either hyper (too much ass) or hypo (flat ass), then you have the perfect condition for back troubles. Take note that hyper is the better option of the two. Better, but still painful, and not even remotely as common as the hypos sitting around out there.

PERFECT CURVE

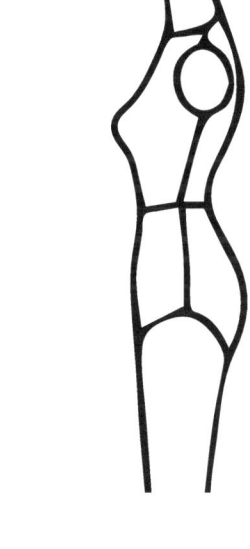

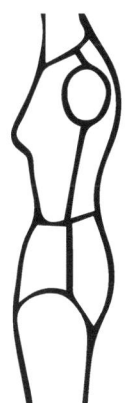

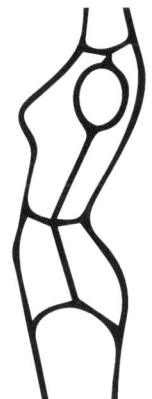

Hypolordosis   Hyperlordosis

SPINE DESIGN

The design of the lumbar spine is an amazing thing. When stacking one bone on top of the other, Lego-block style, you will create a c-shaped, half moon, banana shaped form. It's your natural curve and any deviation from this bony position is termed "ab"-normal.

The theory behind standing erect and developing all these windy back curves—as seen from a side view position—is to smooth your gait. The windy curves give you shock absorption power, allowing for two things: you can withstand high loads and you don't walk like you've dropped an accidental load in your pants. Ever had a lift in the back of an old pick-up truck? No springs, no backseat, and lots of height from the tiniest of bumps! There are other reasons why we develop s-curves once we get up on our feet, but the balance and shock absorption theories are the strongest and most interesting ones. Remember, I promised to keep things simple!

The next anatomical concepts to grasp are the "bone-disc-bone" and "bone-bone" relationships, together, and with each other. How do these stacked-up bones work together to help you bend over to pet the cat...or not?

Pretend your hand is one independent vertebral bone. Place one hand on top of the other, palms together and parallel to the ground—like you would if you were holding a cup of coffee with one hand holding onto the bottom of the cup and the other on top. Next, place an imaginary jelly donut in between your fingers. Only the fingers get to hold the donut. Your palms are touching skin-on-skin. There you have it: the perfect vertebral complex simulation model. A vertebral complex is made up of two independent vertebral bones interacting together in an anatomical partnership. These complex couples start from the very base of your lumbar spine and run all the way up to your head. Whenever you pick two vertebrae, any two, you have a vertebral complex. A stack makes a column; hence, the phrase "spinal column". A motor unit (motor means movement) is the same as a vertebral complex.

How do these complex partnerships get along? Well, are you still holding the donut? The front part (fingers-donut-fingers) is the bone-disc-bone part of the complex. The palm-to-palm, or skin-on-skin. contact represents the bone-to-bone contact. Your fingers are pointing forward, so the finger-donut-finger part is the front part of the complex. The palm-to-palm contact represents the back part of the complex. Don't get sweaty palms over this spatial description. Backbones have front (a.k.a. anterior) and back (a.k.a. posterior) parts. Next, spread your thumbs and little pinkies apart. These represent the bony winged extensions of the vertebral complex. These bony wings provide a place for ligaments and muscles to attach. Now move your hands up and down, swish them side-to-side, point up toward the sky and point downward toward the ground, carefully, so as not to create any turbulence in the Air Donut's jelly compartment. Chef Rice welcomes you. Have a safe bite!

A BOY STAR IS BORN

There is another way to describe the seven essential parts of a vertebra. Looking at a vertebra from a superior (above) view it looks like a star. Draw a regular star using five straight lines the way you were taught in grade school— you know, the star you can draw without lifting the pen off the paper. Next, draw another star, but this time around, flatten the top point of your star. On this second flat-headed star, draw an extra point between the star's two legs…kind of like making it into a boy star. Make the boy star point (the middle leg) twice as long as the other ones. You now have a six-pointed star with a flat head. Number the top flat head of the star as number one. Moving clockwise, number all six star parts. The pentagon-shaped center of the star can be number seven.

Number one, the vertebral body, is the front part of the vertebra. The donut disc sits between two vertebral bodies. The donut discs are jelly-like in the center and have a surrounding wall of webbed fibers to make sure the jelly stays fresh in its inside compartment.

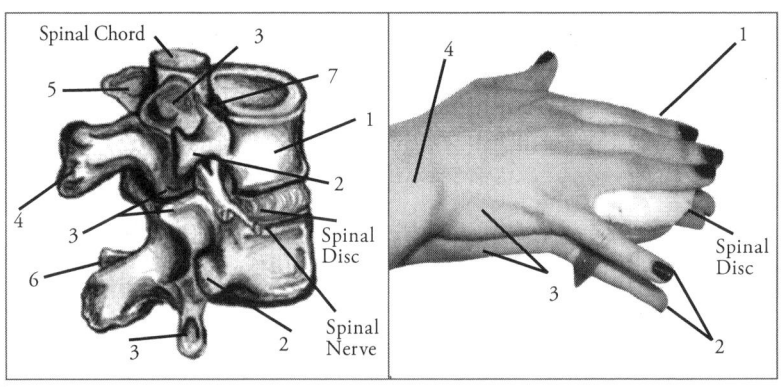

"bone-disc-bone" & "bone-bone" relationships

Numbers two and six are the "transverse processes." These are the thumb and pinky wings of Air Donut. "Transverse" means it is positioned sideways, and "process" means something's sticking out, as in when his process is transverse, you know he's enjoying the view of your lordotic curves.

Numbers three and five are the facet joints. If two stars are placed one on top of the other, forming a vertebral complex, the pair of threes and fives form a facet joint. This type of joint is a bone-on-bone joint just like your finger joints. Lubricated by synovial (see-no-evil) fluid, they slide smoothly on each other. Synovial fluid is like Ma Nature's very own WD-40. These same facet joints help stop you from making an ass of yourself by preventing you from bending over backwards too far.

Number four is a favorite of mine, the spinous process— just another process that points straight back. These are the bones you can actually touch and feel in a person's back. In some people, when looking at their backs, you can actually see their spinous processes...little bumps running all the way up their back.

Number seven is a dead space, an empty space, an imaginary hole called the vertebral canal. A canal is created if you stack a whole bunch of vertebrae one on top of the other. This tunnel is home and protection for your cord. This nerve train-track, called the spinal cord, starts at the base of your brain and runs in the tunnel right through to your butt. The examination of our body's inner beauty is now complete. Hopefully, it was love at first sight!

The spinal column has three components: **the spinal stack, the nerves and the muscles.**

1. MY MY, WHAT BIG BONES YOU HAVE!

Your backbone is the framework of your being—star-shaped lumbar vertebrae stacked one on top of the other, creating a dipping lordosis, a perfect five star stack that produces a tunnel of protection against life's blows.

2. MY OH MY, THAT FEELS GREAT

How else could you know how good things feel if it weren't for your nerves? They exit between each vertebra and follow specific paths that are as complicated as the New York subway. The nerve paths go to your groin parts, to your waistline, to your gut, and down your legs. The nerves supply power to your muscles, to your internal organs, to your skin (no nerves, no pain AND no pleasure). Nerves have ports of exit located between each vertebra, between star points two and three on the right, and five and six on the left. If anything goes wrong in the vicinity, nerves talk back...and if you have pain you now know where some of them go. That cramp in your muscle is your nerves' way of telling you there's a blockage in the vicinities of boy star numbers two-three or five-six!

3. MY, WHAT BIG MUSCLES YOU HAVE

Contracting muscles cause movement. Ligaments, like duct tape, hold everything together and assist in keeping your movements smooth. Bones hold bodies erect, but it is muscles and ligaments that keep you standing through the pressures of your environment.

Keep in mind that your upper spine has other functions too, such as standing in as a comfort attachment zone for

A STAR IS BORN

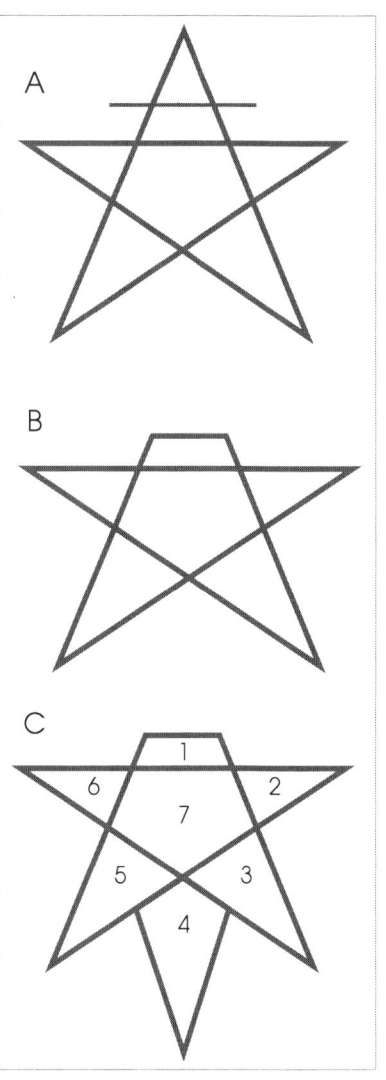

THE SEVEN ESSENTIAL PARTS OF A VERTEBRA

1. Vertebral body
2. Transverse processes
3. Facet joints
4. Spinous process
5. Facet joints
6. Transverse processes
7. Vertebral canal

your chest's ribs. Looking past the superficiality of bulging "pecs" and deep cleavage, your ribs provide protection for more important body parts like those vital organs called heart and lungs! To examine the inner body, Leonardo da Vinci performed 30 human dissections. For me five was enough. You, on the other hand, just have to remember to thank those who have graciously given their bodies for the advancement of spinal research and development...yours!

5

LOVE STORY

Now let us take a moment to go from the dynamics of the inner body to the scary aerodynamics of the outer body. Meet Jack and Jill, new lovers with disturbing symptoms.

Jill, "Ouch!"
Jack, "Sorry!"
"OUCH!"
"WHAT?"
"You're really hurting me!"
Jack explains, "Well…you're really tight in there!"
"I'm tight in there? You're rough in there!"
"You're too sensitive! I'm hardly touching you!"
Jill replies, "Well, in my book, you're still too rough. Go easy or I won't let you show me."

"You're the one who agreed to try this."

"And I only agreed to let you show me how you do it because I don't believe you're as good as you say you are!"

"You see? I just knew you needed it bad. If this is too rough for you…"

"Ohhh! Jack…"

"I'm not giving up on you. All you need is a little bit more. Stay with me, babe. Let me…move…into…this spot. Feel anything?"

"Does annoyed count? Oh wait! Let me spread my leg out a bit, my hips are cramping this way."

"Feel this spot?"

Jill yells, "Oh yeah!"

"See how it makes your back arch? Yeah…Baby! When your head tilts back like that…your mouth all open like that…eyes all rolled up in your head. This is feeling goooood. Let's cool it a bit, people are beginning to notice."

"Oh yeah, it's happening, I tell ya! Don't stop! I should pay you to make me feel this good."

"I'd let you buy me a drink but I think we just closed the bar again!"

"Any refreshments at your house?"

"As much as my bar fridge will hold."

"Let's go! That's one bar we're not gonna get kicked out of tonight! But I'll only go on one condition, though."

"Pick up where we left off?"

"This time, Jack, the pantyhose are coming off. Damn that foot massage of yours…it's kingdom come!"

So how many times has a possible lover tried to show you his or her performance as a lover by giving you a little massage? It's the oldest trick in the book. Don't fall for it. A quickie massage is no way to get the measure of a lover's abilities.

Alas they never listen. Jill is a woman of risk and adventure, yet she can be tense and full of resistance. Tonight, she feels unusually comfortable with this man called Jack. She is excited about Jack's invitation to play.

Jack, on the other hand, is excitable yet smoothly submissive. He gets touchy-feely after the initial inhibition-releasing effect of his first drink has kicked in. Tonight, the conversation was light and lucky.

"I'm Jack."
"I'm Jill."
"What's up?"
"My bill."
"If I pay the tab, will you raise a little hell with me?"
"If you pay the tab, I will raise a little leg with you!"

He shoots, he scores! Her posture sways. She's sore!

Tonight Jill's suffocating in her pretty little dress. With this in mind she's purposely orchestrating her quick 'getting to know you' session with Jack. He's being set up for a good time with only Jill's selfish good intentions in mind. Jack's not so different. His good intention is to have a good time and show off while he's at it. He's the man with a plan!

Jill listens to her body. She knows what she needs to keep her from feeling she's over the hill. Her back pain always clears up after a successful Jack-fetching chase. So tonight Jill's hiking path leads her to climb right to the top of the hill to fetch her a Jack to jump in the sack. All she hopes for now is that Jack is functional enough to help her unscrew her chronically painful and contorted back. Jill seduces Jack the way she shops for shoes. Forget price— she's attracted to looks and durability.

What Jill doesn't know, because she skipped the Sisy Squat Sex Test, is that Jack has broken his crown once or twice in the past. Many of you are familiar with his medical history. A trip here, a bump there, some undiagnosed low back disc wear and tear. Unfortunately, in Jack's case his injury has quickly ripened into degenerative arthritis.

Watch your step, Jill. The front steps of Jack's trailer are steeper than expected. This place is so small that you can hear Jill's thought: "…not even enough room for an imaginary friend." Ouch! Jack is proud of his pad. Once inside, they sit side-by-side on the narrow and thin-cushioned sofa bed. Watch your back, Jackass.

Jill wastes no time. She has a mission. They start standing. As soon as she wraps her legs around his waist, he sees all kinds of stars—big bright ones floating around his visual field, and shooting flaming ones with long tails traveling fast all the way down his right leg. The shooting ones were especially prickly to feel, running from his buttock to his Achilles' heel.

"Star light-Star bright — Why did my back have to break tonight?" he moans.

"I can't stand it!" he yells.

"You don't want to do this?"

"No, I can't stand it anymore!"

Jill tries to understand again. "You don't like doing it this way?"

"No, I just can't," he mutters back.

That wasn't it at all. Poor Jack just can't stand up anymore.

Well, that's probably the end of Jack's one-night stand. Doesn't look like Jill is going to climb any hills tonight. Poor Jill, if only she had done a test run on the merchandise. If only she had Jack do the Sisy Squat Sex Test on him before saying yes to Jack's invitation. And poor, painful Jack the sap.

6

THE DETERMINATORS:
FINAL JUDGMENT

You rush to the emergency room in acute distress. Shooting pain slicing your body in two makes death look like a promising cure! Unless a knife can be seen sticking out from your lumbars, doctors must uncover your determinators (causes) to classify your pain, and, yes, you will be instructed to "bend over to touch your toes" for a rear view gawk of your hump and an unintentional gape of your rump.

Back injuries are classified into broad categories. These categories define "the broken back." Each broad category is an E.R. nickname describing both the main tissues involved in the patient's pain and describing the patient's physical problem. The E.R. nicknames have many specific dysfunctions, syndromes, and disease sub-categories within them.

It's a busy night in the E.R.. Examination rooms are not packed with the typical drunken brawlers; they're packed with "spinals." Privacy curtains are closed, patients are moaning louder than an all-male colonoscopy examination room, and bodies are fidgeting into less-pained horizontal poses. Charts hang in their wall baskets, identifying the patient name, medical history, and possible determinator factors. E.R. residents get ready for their introductions. The patients are well-identified by their ID bracelets.

In the E.R. and on the examination table, placing the patient in the correct spinal diagnostic category is the most important initial teamwork task to perform. The questioning, the examining, the poking, the testing, and sometimes, the blood sucking will, hopefully, yield the identity of what is causing the back pain. Determining the category in which the spinal diagnostic fits into is the first step in fixing the problem.

CALLING PATIENT MICK ANNICKLE

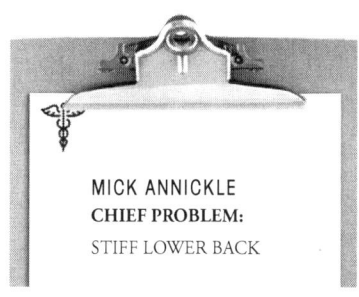

MICK ANNICKLE
CHIEF PROBLEM:
STIFF LOWER BACK

Patient Mick Annickle's problem is of a biomechanical nature. (Bio, as in biology, and mechanical, as in gears and chains). He's been told he's a "mechanopath." Unknown to him, his friends call him "stiffy," and not in a good way! A diesel mechanic for five years, Mick's heavy lifting is taking a toll on his low back. He should count himself blessed for the early detection and warning sign of a mechanically malfunctioning backbone. Mechanopaths are laden with bones that will not go where the mechanopaths want them to go. The bones are either stuck or, worse, stuck in the wrong place. They are simply not going anywhere the mechanopath wants to go. Predictably, they stay right where they are as the mechanopath moves about.

So if you are the mechanopath, then off you go back home. But first, you will have to stop to fill the pharmaceutical prescription you were given. The chef at Chez Pharmo has prepared a petite yet very palatable three-course medi-meal just for you. You will be served a stiff non-alcoholic aperitif of muscle relaxant with lime-flavored spring water. The water will help flush the relaxant down. For the entrée, a mindaltering serving of analgesics will be served. Finally, you will need a good body mechanic to help fix your bent-out-of-shape state. Yes, you can go home but you have homework.

CALLING PATIENT MIA PATTO

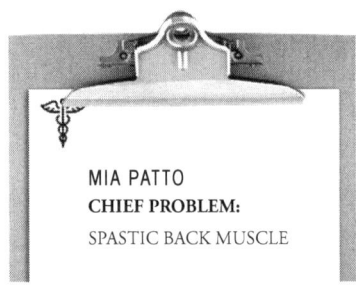

MIA PATTO
CHIEF PROBLEM:
SPASTIC BACK MUSCLE

The patient in the room next to the mechanopath is ready. Her long hours at the car assembly plant have brought her sore back into the E.R. No matter how often she circulates job tasks, an unbearable soreness always settles in by the end of her day. Today, she cannot take it anymore.

Residents have labeled her chart as being in the myopa-thology category of spinal problems. Her friends have cun-ningly labeled her a "spaz"! Mia has been labeled as being a "myopath." Fear not, she's not the most complicated patient in the E.R., but that doesn't mean that Mia is not experiencing a great deal of pain. The myopath patient is easy to diagnose because her source of back pain—a tight spastic support muscle—is sometimes visible, and it is always touchable.

Sometimes myopathic problems accompany other, more important categories. A thorough E.R. resident will always investigate further to eliminate the possibility of a more complicated underlying condition the myopath may be hiding.

On the other extreme side of a spasmodic myopathic condi-tion is its opposite form. The opposite is a weakened and wasted back muscle that will contribute as much mechanical malfunc-tion as a spastic one. This problem also fits into the "myopath" category of back problems. It's not, however, Miss Mia's problem!

The myopath patient is likely a repeat visitor to the E.R., always with the same complaint. Chances are high that the muscle texture is changing with every acute episodic back attack. Recurrences turn "myo" toward the "pathic" direction and transform the muscle texture into a non-edible, grizzled back steak that would intimidate even Hannibal Lector.

So if you are the myopath then off you go but first, you too will have to make a stop to fill the prescription you were given in the E.R. On this visit, the chef at Chez Pharmo recommends a spa-like diet feast. You will be given a warm-up cocktail of ergogenic (which means fat burner) caffeinated extra-hot latte with a fair sized-sprinkle of powdered muscle relaxant topping that extra foam. Then you will be encouraged to participate in the spa-like exercise therapy: mobilization (someone electrifies you up, down and all around), massage (someone kneads you around), passive stretching (someone pulls you around), and physical therapy (someone electrifies you).

CALLING PATIENT SUE WELLINGS

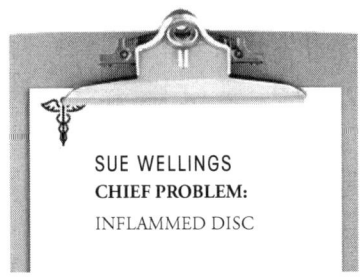

SUE WELLINGS
CHIEF PROBLEM:
INFLAMMED DISC

The emergence of deep swelling in the disc and other surrounding tissues has brought Ms. Sue Wellings into the E.R., because she was convinced this pain was not going to go away on its own. A juvenile court attorney, she's worried about these recurrent bouts of low back pain, especially because all she does is sit, dictate, and bill all day. The lingo outlined on the chart will read "inflammatory something or another." Sue Wellings is sore and her chart reads "inflammopath." Her friends sympathetically call her "Puffy." What Sue Wellings feels is as painful as the word "inflammation" sounds. Damaged discs, either by herniation, bulging, or tearing, are swollen. A degenerated disc is also very likely susceptible to acute recurring bouts of inflammation.

Her file may be flagged for an emergency consultation with the staff neurosurgeon. The surgeon may then request an M.R.I. (Magnetic Resonance Imaging) scan. This costly imaging format may be warranted for a better picture of

50

the disc status. The warranted facts, however, may still not bump you up on the M.R.I. waiting list. If Sue screams loud enough (from the ache and not the lousy appointment date she was given for the M.R.I. scan) she may be bumped up from the average three-month waiting time. On the somber side for the inflammopath, if damages are discal in nature, they may be permanent.

So if you are the inflammopath, on your way out of the E.R. you will have to make a stop to fill the pharmaceutical prescription you were given. On this visit, the chef at Chez Pharmo will feed you a filling portion of "antis": anti-swelling, anti-welting, anti-pain, and anti-worsening. The anti-inflammatory pills will stop the swelling progression and help heal the tissues that are all puffed up. Although it is doubtful that icing will penetrate deep enough to have a direct "Mr. Freeze" effect on the deep swollen tissues, ice is still good to flush out local blood pooling and put a temporary stop to the wailing temperament of local neurons.

Three down and two suffering spines to go! So far, we have successfully identified the problems of the first three patients and have discharged them from the E.R.: Patient "Mick the Mechanopath" with a mechanical back bone problem; patient "Mia the Myopath" with tough and tight back muscles; and patient "Sue the Inflammopath" with a swollen low back disc. Their charts have been put away, their health insurance numbers have been recorded, and off they go to Chez Pharmo. Two more curtain calls are left for our examining, diagnosing and prescriptive call.

CALLING PATIENT N. ERV STENSION

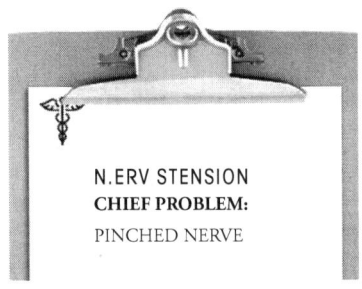

N.ERV STENSION
CHIEF PROBLEM:
PINCHED NERVE

The E.R. lingo associated with Erv's suffering is neuropathology and his file says "neuropath." Spinal nerves get involved because they can be victims of stretching, pressure, choking, or clogging abuse. In Erv's case his spinal nerves have been choked by long car rides on stiff lumbar discs. If it were brain nerves involved, Erv would be wheeled up to psychiatry. Since spinal nerves are the tissues involved, however, the neuropath, as opposed to psycho, may be wheeled up to neurology.

Neuropathology is a complicated category and the neuropath is a complicated patient. His friends call him "Sparky" and they don't mean to compliment him! Symptoms of a neuropath will make their presence known elsewhere, far from the original problem, like deep down into the legs, all the way down to your tippy toes. Wherever the nerves go, the pain flows!

N. Erv Stension is a challenging patient to the E.R. resident. The resident will call for a neuro-surgical consultation, especially if the patient's pain is accompanied by other spinal diagnostic categories (inflammopath, myopath, mechanopath). It will ultimately be the call of the neuro-medical experts to determine if there is a need to order imaging pictures beyond radiographs. When dealing with neuropaths, a lot of pictures may be involved but I can assure you, this is one photo shoot you want to avoid.

So if you are the suffering neuropath, off you go for your pharmaceutical prescription. Your prescription will likely be a temporary and tightly controlled fill of analgesics kept under lock and key. Analgesics should keep the pain at bay until you can be further assessed by your private primary care practitioner. Your primary care practitioner will very likely recommend four things: a nerve conduction test, another consult with a neurologist, more behind-the-counter nerve-sitting pills, and a good mechanosis body shop. You will become very familiar with Chez Pharmo as a frequent visitor.

CALLING PATIENT ART WRIGHTESS

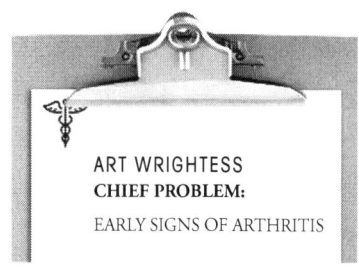

ART WRIGHTESS
CHIEF PROBLEM:
EARLY SIGNS OF ARTHRITIS

Art Wrightess is well acquainted with the E.R. His condition has brought him there many times. Mr. Wrightess built almost all of the stone fireplaces in his town. He's known to his clients as "Creaky" but the keywords in the E.R. are "degenerative arthropathology." Bony growths, decay and scarring that fuse the body prevent smooth action. He has no hope to ever move well again. His condition will cause a chronically collapsing nervous system. Decaying bones, scarred surrounding tissue, and dysfunctional local nerve tissue are marked characteristics of the "Golden Generation!"

Art Wrightess is an "arthropath." Arthropath comes from arthro-joint and pathy-not healthy. He will be sent to radiology for bone pictures. Once the severity of decay has been determined, Art will very likely be referred for a rheumatology consultation. When decaying bones alter nerve function, they may cause other body system malfunctions.

So if you are the suffering degenerative arthropath, you too will need a pharmaceutical prescription. The addition of prescriptive medicine for the arthropath is hardly a change to a senior's daily intake schedule. The average senior will consume approximately five different medical remedies. Your table has been reserved at Chez Pharmo for some time. You'll be served up a smorgasbord of anti-inflammatories and killers of pain, and a muscle relaxant may be up for grabs. The long-term plan is to keep moving and exercise daily.

CURTAIN CALL

The E.R. is finally empty! Following the determinator identification step, a classification arrangement by tissue type and then simplifying the E.R. lingo, the broad categories of low back problems can be arranged as follows:

The Stiffy Mechanopath = Mick Annickle (think mechanical)

The Spazzy Myopath = Mia Patto (think muscle)

The Puffy Inflammopath = Sue Wellings (think swelling)

The Sparky Neuropath = N. Erv Stension (think nerve)

The Creaky Arthropath = Art Wrightess (think arthritis)

To understand these five broad categories is a big leap forward in the subject of lumbar anatomical, determinator, and diagnostic groupings. Congratulations! You have passed the basics of a back education program. You have been picked as a Survivor.

7

THE DETERMINATORS
OR THE GATHERING OF
YOUR IMPERFECTIONS

I have coined a word to describe the causes of back pain. "Determinators" are the factors that contribute to your pain. Identifying determinators helps point to a complete diagnosis of back pain. What causes your pain? Too much exercise? Weakness brought on by heredity? The physical stresses of parenting? Or the physical stresses of partying? The reason a person has back pain can help fix the problem. If you're lucky, removing the back pain cause will remove the pain and prevent recurrences. If sitting on your wallet all day long causes your back pain, for example, then stay off that wallet and it won't come back.

If back pain recurs it is often more intense the second and third times around. It used to be good enough to receive back pain advice, like, "Take two of these and call me in the morning." "If it hurts, don't do it!" "Stay off your feet for a few days." "Read this pamphlet, do the exercises every day, and take the rest of the week off." Back pain is more complex and more serious than that old advice suggests. The determinator is an unknown dark force. Most patients claim to have been doing nothing at the time back pain appeared. Some will admit they were performing the simplest "coming" activity when their pain appeared: they were coming out of the shower, coming out of the car, coming off the toilet, coming back up from picking up a gym bag, or quite simply, just coming and going.

EXPLAINING THE PAIN

The science of figuring out the determinators that cause the pain is Etiology. The long list of etiological determinators is usually grouped into very general categories, such as mechanical, stress, and systemic but as you might expect, my version of this list is based on my real life practice. In no particular order of importance the determinators of back pain are:

1. Sexual Absenteeism
2. Body Mechanic Determinators
    i. Bad Ass-titude— Posture
    ii. Back Luck— Trauma
    iii. Repeat Yourself— Repetitive Strain
    iv. What Lies Beneath—Pelvic & Leg Problems
    v. Seat Yourself —Sitting on Your Ass
    vi. Pleas of Innocence: Inexplicable Mechanosis & Inexplicable Occurrence
3. Deep Thoughts Deep Pain— The Stress Determinators

4. The Systemic Determinators
5. The Hoola Scoop
6. The Degenerate Determinator

1. SEXUAL ABSENTEEISM

Sex can be the healing medicine for the ninety percent of us who will get low back pain. "When was the last time you got it?" "Hmm!" As chicken soup is to the common cold, a roll in the sack is to the sexually suffocated spine. And please note, sex not only prevents back pain, it also helps cure back pain.

2. THE BODY MECHANIC DETERMINATORS

When statistical findings suggest that ninety percent of us will get the low back plague at least once in our lives, it is very likely what I call "spinal mechanosis" or malfunction that they are talking about. Ninety percent of us will have a mechanical breakdown that will cause back pain.

I have categorized spinal mechanosis into six sub-categories, but before carrying on with further introductions to the mechanosis family members, here is a brief explanation of what mechanosis involves:

Mechanical body functions are termed "altered" or "dysfunctional" when joint motion becomes irregular or painfully odd. Remembering the previously described vertebral motor unit, (two vertebrae moving together— any two will do), when a complex loses its ability to move along one of its designated planes of motion (bend forward, arch back, rotate right or lean left…), spinal mechanosis has occurred, and low back pain soon follows. It's the beginning of mechanosis.

The inability of a motor unit to move smoothly will result in pain in and around the area of dysfunction. Attempts to drive the body in directions prohibited by joint mechanical malfunctions result in the basis of mechanosis: impaired driving! You turn the steering wheel to the right, but the wheels go left or don't move at all!

Causes of mechanosis vary because of everyone's individuality—to each his own. Mechanosis is the consequential physical expression of your "self". They are irreproducible! They express your unique physique. They are your very own spinal imprints, like your thumb's curvilinear graphic art! Looking into the causes of mechanosis expression, I have assembled the following mechanosis commonalities: I) Bad Ass-titude—Posture, II) Bad Luck—Trauma, III) Repeat Your Self—Repetitive Strain, IV) What Lies Beneath—Pelvic and Leg Problems, V) Seat Your Self—Sitting On Your Ass, and VI) Pleas of Innocence—Doin' Nothin' and Hurtin' Somethin' Bad.

I) BAD ASS-TITUDE—POSTURE

You wake up one morning, look in the mirror and say, "Hell, what happened to my posture?" Glad you finally noticed! After all, every posture says a thousand words. Let it be known that attitude with bad posture has mechanosis consequences—hence, the birth of your "bad ass-titude"! Expressively holding yourself in positions other than what are considered "normal anatomical positions," like equal pelvic level with normal dipping lumbar curves, will have mechanosis consequences. Be aware or beware the spinal wear!

Then there's the brain game. Here's an awakening experimental visual thrill for you: get naked, look in the mirror, and hold yourself up tall—like you're walking the runway, modeling underpants. Is it your rippling muscular strength that is fashioning a positive impact on your present as-good-as-it-gets conscientious stance, or is it your eye message to your brain, telling your muscles

EVERY POSTURE SAYS A THOUSAND WORDS

to change their contractibility to improve how you look, standing there before your nakedness, waiting for your audience to applaud? For most of us, it's a brain game we have to play in order to improve those bad ass-titude postures we hold all day long. Remember, your brain plays an important role in your posture.

You want to look good in your new clothes, so you stand tall. You get out of the dressing room to see what the new khakis look like, so you stand tall, chest out, in front of a mirror for a self-examination. Then, you carry on with life outside the change room mirror and stop playing The Brain Game. You slouch, you swagger, and you swish. Remember this lesson: Use brain…avoid cane. No brain…no posture. Bad ass-titude…bad back! Those are The Brain Game rules!

Posture–Breathing–Thinking: those are the rules of meditation. You see, thinking and posture go hand-in-hand. The Yogi's ten-hour meditation marathons of posture–breathing–thinking awaken a message to the brain that says, "Better posture improves health and thinking." This message will shape up the structural posture muscles.

Has your inner Buddha gong rung yet? Will the way your brain carries your "self" be improved? Do you think you can be a good brain game player? Rest assured that it does not take a ten hour Yogi session to improve your posture. It only takes a mere brain game awakening moment to remind yourself that many times during the day, you're not holding yourself well. Remember that people are still watching you, even if you're not doing the runway thing! There's always someone watching! Hold yourself well. Imagine ten hours of posture–breathing–thinking! Ouch...my poor knees! I don't know about you, but I prefer posture–breathing–eating, followed by posture–breathing–napping! That's the French way!

II) BAD LUCK—TRAUMA

Accidental falls and tragic mishaps cause altered skeletal mechanosis. Earth's powerful g-forces on your falling bones, the leverage forces of your free-falling long bones, the asymmetrically sustained g-forces on any back bone, the sudden accelerating forces on your otherwise silent and unmoving bones, the sudden decelerating forces on your moving bones...they hurt joints and rip muscles. They create mechanosis! They create severe insult to the spine. Tough "lock" for you!

LET HER RIP

When we overextend ourselves we introduce the g-forces of nature that cause sprains and strains. Strains occur when muscles or tendons are stretched beyond their limits.

Furthermore, the overstretched tissues will usually cause your muscles to spastically tighten up. This, believe it or not, is supposed to be protection against further injury—more disabling pain! Thanks! If left untreated, the chronic spasms develop triggers—not the happiest g-spot on your body. These muscle g-spots create even more pain when touched or stretched.

Sprains occur when ligaments overstretch or rip. Think of ligaments as bone-to-bone humanoid duct tape, but spines are not spandex stretch-proof. Bending way over, butt in the air position, and ready for pick up ("Oh golly, my shoelace keeps getting untied…you think he was looking this time?"), your muscles are in a relaxed-mode, and your ligaments are in their "stretched-and-ready-to-rip" mode. Perhaps visibly appealing (He was watching after all!), it still remains an anatomically vulnerable position. Gymnasts, Northwestern cheerleaders, and Angelina Jolie are exempted from this rule! Ready to rip one, or two for that matter, twisting or coming back up not empty-handed will be the cause of tissue failure, which will either keep you in the butt-up stuck position, or quickly push you into the nasty floor dive.

III) REPEAT YOUR SELF—REPETITIVE STRAIN

You repeat yourself too much! Say what? Repeat yourself! Repeat myself? No, repeat yourself! Repeat yourself? Yes! Me? I give up!

Repeating yourself is not only painful for you; it can also be painful for others, too. Every day and in so many ways, we show in the actions of our everyday routines signs and symptoms of suffering from "Excessive Compulsive Disorder." Day in and day out, in and out, back and forth, wax-on wax-off, you put your right foot in and then your right foot out, open and close, lift and lower, see-saw, up and down, clockwise counter-clockwise, rub-on rub-off, twist-on twist-off, take-in take-off, put-on take-off... check-in too much, and you're likely to check-out with some over-utilized, tired, burned-out, and inflamed spinal tissues. Call it the "robo-mechanosis." Robotic movements eventually impair the body's overly-"roboticized" joints, which lead to repetitive mechanosis. Are you a "roboholic" workaholic, or are you just plain dedicated to your work?

IV) WHAT LIES BENEATH—PELVIC AND LEG PROBLEMS

The concept that what lies beneath is capable of affecting your performance can be explained using that overprotected "designated parking spot" problem of yours. You're late for work, you want to park the car in your special designated spot, and someone is parked in it. That selfish bastard... doesn't he know you have high blood pressure? So instead of using your car blocking modus operandi (didn't work the last time, the bastard still got away), or key-scratching instructions on his door telling him where to park next time (not good...this is just not a good idea), you opt for your third modus operandi: take someone else's spot. So you've now set the pattern for a domino effect—a good example of a nasty chain reaction. The negativity moves onto the spot next to you, and the next guy will very likely park in the spot next to the one you just took, and so on, and so on. Going back to blocking back bones, if you have an illegally blocking mechanosis down there, below your belt, the problem will quickly be spread to another parking spot, mainly the next articulation above and below your designated parking spot!

Hits below the belt cause mechanosis above and below the spot that's been hit. What lies below your low back area are possible hidden mechanosis factors that will tip off the normalcy of your bony motor units by tipping off your bone balance. Think: "bottoms-up"! What lies beneath are physical individualities that may also make their presence known upabove, in your lumbar spine: physical beauty marks like a tipping short leg (short leg, as in "get me another chair, this one rocks when I sit on it," or maybe you're more familiar with the folded napkin underneath the leg of a table?), an altered strut, caved-in Daffy Duck paws, rubbing knock-knees, pointing pigeon toes, riding cowboy legs, sexy butt wiggles, and tight, knotty ass and leg muscles. The beauty of our physical individualities may hold costly mechanosis consequences.

V) SEAT YOUR SELF—SITTING ON YOUR ASS

Seat yourself first, and then help yourself to a big-assed portion of mechanosis. Sitting is the worst of bad postural habits, and the vilest of mechanosis poisoning. Man may thinketh, but why doth he hast to do so in a sitteth position? We are architecturally designed to stand; our sitting habit is a mechanosis etiology not to ignore! More on this later, as sitting deserves a standing ovation all of its own for "Best Performing Determinator."

OLD SCHOOL SERGEANTS—CHIEF COMMANDERS OF CHAIR-SITTERS

Remember your grade school chairs—the ones with a thin band of plastic or pressed plywood resting horizontally on your tiny shoulder blades? Remember your teacher with the mammoth head, big hair, big hands, firm grip, and super long, pointy, pokey, bossy fingers? Remember the teacher commands to sit up straight? How many times were you told, "You can't learn if you slouch!" (Yeah, right!) "Your shoulders will stay like that if you don't sit up!" (The teach was right about this one!) For every long distance gawk, and for every supervisory aisle walk, you straightened up and held up as long as the teacher was looking. If sitting up was so good for you, then why was it so hard to stay up in the first place? Why was it so difficult to concentrate on schoolwork when forced to sit up straight? Why didn't they make it easier for our little bodies to sit up straight? Was a shoulder tap or back poke supposed to be enough support to make things easier for us?

SLOUCHING
KILLS BONERS

The academic commanders wanted us all to be chairperson candidates for the "Society of the Straight Spine Sitters." How could the scary, big-faced Commanding Generals of our Grade School Platoon not see that we could not possibly hold this position long enough to not get caught slouching? We were mere little chair-people of the "Society of Scholastic Slouchers"—helpless little slouchers!

Your throne is hurting your bones! And you can blame your pain on the design fault of your lumbar bones. It's a sad thing to favor resting on our sit-upon, even if the design is faulty and a danger to low back stability. We sit all day and wonder why our bad backs are forever violating their parole. Medical officers stand guard, trying to rescue us from our long history of ignorance and abuse.

To better understand this all-too-common determinator, we need to address some important sitting facts. Our low back is the main load-bearing wall of our spine. Sitting compromises the bearing wall for three reasons. One, as the load position shifts to a different location, our center of gravity changes accordingly. Two, our pelvis is flexed (a forward tilting pelvis, the position your pelvis takes on when someone's just punched you in the stomach, changes the load location, too). Three, our psoas muscle is strained (shortened and tightened). The psoas is a back muscle that attaches itself on your hips. For Hannibals, it's the filet mignon of the human body. Watch out, Clarice Starling!

When sitting, the bending moment (a dark force that wants to collapse you in half) shifts forward. This is a place that isn't ready to unconditionally accept the loving weight of your upper body. Conditions of pain, bulging discs, and progressive spinal decay apply. And sadly, this is only the beginning.

STANDOFFISH AND STANDING TALL

We are designed to be standing upright. Upright means low disc pressure. Low disc pressure means happy disc stability. The low back discs are most stable in the lordotic position. Sitting is the least favorite position because the normal hollow in the low back, the lordosis, is collapsed. A flattened low back is an invitation to bulging discs and stretched ligaments, amongst other things.

What becomes, then, of our chronically sitting selves? Since sitting is the enemy position, those who succumb to the grueling bending moment that turns lordotic to alordotic eventually become "disclexics." Disclexics are suffering souls carrying the sins of a mechanosis-infected spine. Disclexics suffer because they are spastic, bulging, and decaying fast.

THROWING YOU OFF YOUR SEAT

Here's something to sit and think about, a concept to challenge your understanding of the sitting principles just discussed. When sitting on a stool, keeping your lordosis alive requires a tremendous amount of muscular activity. After a while, you get tired and let the heavy weight of your upper body take over, pulling you into a position that requires less muscle contraction energy. A position called "the slouch!"

The slouch is a more relaxed sitting pose. It requires little muscle energy expenditure. This minimal muscle contraction energy is enough, luckily, to at least keep you from falling over like you're in the airplane crash position. On the other hand, slouching, you already know, steps your bones down from a favorable lordotic c-curve to a less favorable alordotic position, which means that lumbar disc pressure increases, lumbar mechanics become dysfunctional, and a wear pattern follows suit. Damned if you keep your lordosis unsupported, and damned if you don't! So what is there to think about? This thought illustrates that you actually don't need muscle activity to degenerate. You can actually decay away just by sitting around. Yes, the slouching helps reduce the muscle load, but the new bone position encourages degeneration. You just can't win! So the lesson to learn is clear: slouching kills boners.

How, then, can you hold the proper lordotic c-curve while at the same time satisfying the need to minimize the contractile forces of your back muscles? Easy: with an outside back up, of course! The right thing to do is to use an outside, non-compressible helper that will take over the job of your muscles to hold the more stable lordotic position of your lumbar spine. Filling the open space between the back of the chair and the skin off your back is how you customize the back support and optimize the bone positions, while at the same time minimizing the muscle strain.

WORLD'S MOST DANGEROUS SEAT

Examining the parts of a toilet seat, you have the hinge joints, and, when in use, you have the weight of your resting ass on the shiny plastic white halo top. The hinge joints are very much like your facet joints (star points three and five articulations with the surrounding stars above and below it). The seat acts like your disc, ready to absorb the pressure of your derriere's weight.

Without your smooth-as-baby's-butt buttock sitting on the toilet disc, the seat will move smoothly and effortlessly. Up and down, for its ladies' and courteous gentlemen's use when bladder pressure urges come upon them. The hinge joints, although receiving the occasional gentleman's uric acid squirt, have no other deteriorating factors that may affect their long-term function of guiding the "toilet seat up–toilet seat down" movements.

When sitting on the toilet "disc", sliding your ass to the side, reaching to grab, perhaps, the sports section of the newspaper on the floor may cause damaging plastic toilet seat cracking and toilet seat hinge stripping. Ouch! The seat will never move the same again. On every sit-upon session, the plastic crack pinches your butt skin on every seat rise and fall, loosened hinges create undesired slipping moments with unnecessary, unwanted crackling noises. The seat has been rendered dysfunctional due to the mechanosis forces of your shearing ass forces—all because you couldn't wait to see how the Yankees did last night. Your every ass-compression sit-down or hinge-pissing stand-up hinge maneuver will worsen the mechanosis problem until, one day, either the seat will no longer welcome derrieres, or the boys will finally have a good reason to be peeing all over that dysfunctional toilet seat.

Sitting on your throne, sofa, lawn chair, or the ground, the "toilet seat injury" phenomena can be compared to the damaging activities on your lumbar disc and facet joints

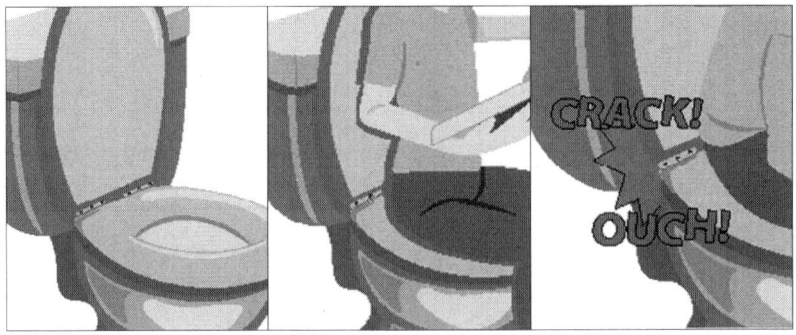

when you sit and twist, together or by themselves! You may never look at your toilet seat the same way again! You also may never want to read the sports section sitting on your ass-halo, either!

VI) PLEAS OF INNOCENCE: INEXPLICABLE MECHANOSIS AND INEXPLICABLE OCCURRENCE

Can you hear the cries of innocence? Were you witness to the innocent playing that caused all the bleeding? Are you a key witness to the bloody move that caused the pain?

Sometimes, the most tranquil postures, the most poised gestures, the most kind-hearted kisses of thanks, and the most childish of play triggers the inexplicable mechanosis. The most well-meaning intentions, the most helpful hands, and the most unexpected acts of kindness can bring up the unexpected mechanosis.

3. DEEP THOUGHTS–DEEP PAIN — THE STRESS DETERMINATORS

"I lay my head down, but the pressure never stops."—2Pac

IF YOU'RE HAPPY AND YOU KNOW IT...

Stressors are factors, not always visible, that create a change in your cool and calm self—a change in your neutral, pH-balanced, rested, and painless state. When stressors change things for the good, we stop calling them stress. Technically, these are called "positive stressors," or eustress. Eustress is defined as a pleasant or curative stress. It is the negative stressors, a.k.a. distress, tipping you into self-destruction or self-defense mode, that we just call "stress". Distress is defined as an unpleasant, disease-producing stress.

Positive or negative, English speakers welcome a wide use of the stress word. It is as popular as the use of the "F" word. As a matter of fact, the "S" word is the new "F" word. The "F" word has a flock of mock expressions that helps show just how one feels in the heat of one's inner moment. The "S" word, like "F", can colorfully express your distress in as many ways as the "F" word. You can be stressed or de-stress. You can stress someone out, be stressless, or stressed to the max. You can stress down, stress about things, be stressing right now, or suffer from post-traumatic stress syndrome. Soon to hit the pop charts of trashy street talk is the recommendation to tell someone who's being incredibly inconsiderate toward your happy and serene inner silence to just "Stress off!" It'll work every time!

Stress is a determinator. There is a physiological explanation for the stress-induced psychosomatic back pain. Changing your neutral pH-balanced brain with a negative stressor will cause hormonal changes in your brain. These changes induce feelings and emotions (fear, anger, hate, frustration, pent-up emotions, depression...), which create chemical reactions in your brain that will cause back spasms. The pain is caused by both a nerve reaction and a chemical reaction from the pro-inflammatory hormones and chemical mediators. The resultant muscle spasms and articular mechanosis will send even more pain messages to your brain. The poor suffering brain will then rev up its message back down to the back muscles and supercharge the spasm. Ouch! I can feel your brain pain now. Well, on the not-so-painful side, this is as much physiology as you need in order to appreciate the "stress-back" pain connection. Enough already!

MAKE-UP AND MAKE-OUT, OR MAKE-OUT AND MAKE-UP?

Situations create feelings that can cause brain chemical reactions. Those physiological stimuli then get into motion and move you right into an immobilizing low back spasm. The best thing to do to break this physiological response of back spasms is to proceed with a therapeutic make-out and make-up session. Erotica can break the neurotica cycles of back pain. This highly recommended therapeutic regimen, hopefully, will clear you of both your negative psychosis (brain nerve problems) and its very close cousin named neurosis (back nerve problems).

FREUDIAN SLIP

Your consciousness, that annoying state of mind you're forced to face in between naps, has the power to help your back pain. Raising the subconscious is how you do it. Psychosomatic back pain evolves from a desire to suppress emotional expression. The result is an expression of the repressed emotion in the soma. Soma, Latin smart talk for body (as opposed to mind), is somewhat smarter than some minds because it does not lie. Your soma does not suppress the pain…it expresses it. He may love you for your soma, but in fact, he could be the cause of your soma pain too! Will you at least think about it?

TOO MUCH LYING AROUND CAN CAUSE SICKLY FEELINGS IN YOUR DORMANT BONES AND RIGID MUSCLES

Amidst all this suppressed soma suffering, there is good news. Conscious awareness that your stress, or someone else's for that matter, could be the cause of your back pain is sometimes enough to fix it altogether. This concept was discussed in "Psycho'-Somatic Medicine." If there is a connection between your back and your stress, and if there is a consciousness there, it is a certainty that having raised the back pain-stress connection into a conscious level is the beginning of healing. That's good news, isn't it? It usually means that you may not need, after all, the weathered buckskin psychiatric chaise lounge to help you deal with your brain pain to help you heal the back pain.

4. THE SYSTEMIC DETERMINATOR—INTERNAL PROGRAMMING CRASH

Systemic back pain is when malfunctioning body parts trick you by making you think the problem's something else, like referring to your back. Sometimes, low back pain is the solo symptom of an illness that has not made its presence known elsewhere. On the other hand, systemic-induced low back pain can present just when you think your other illness can't get any worse. The systemic illness adds yet another symptom to the list of complaints: low back pain. The simultaneous occurrence of back pain with other physical ailments is very common. For some, the back pain may be there simply because the chronic state of spinal immobility, as a result of a bed-ridden illness, has superseded its allowable resting limits. Too much lying around can cause sickly feelings in your dormant bones and rigid muscles.

What illness then, can add onto its symptom repertoire low back pain? There are many on the list, the most common being rheumatoid arthritis, osteoporosis (yes, brittle bones may cause back bone pain), fevers, viral infections, gastro-intestinal problems, kidney disease, bladder infections, gyne-cological problems, and cancers. These maladies are usually medically well cared for. For every ailment listed above, a primary care physician has very likely made the diagnosis, which means that he or she may have also advised of possible systemic-induced back discomfort. The systemic diagnostic will come with advice and a treatment plan that will very likely include care for the accompanying spinal symptom.

When back pain is the solo hint symptom of an underlying systemic malfunction, it is sometimes unfortunate to have overlooked the possibility that the pain is nothing but a sign of trouble elsewhere. Always consider this possibility, always investigate, and like the mammogram, always be assured that the time spent exploring today may give you extra "tomorrow-play."

5. THE HOOLA SCOOP

What great circumferential contours you have...well-defined back muscles, exotic hips, trim pelvic bones, and a non-protuberant, sexy belly. The human hoola hoop is a factor to consider when assessing the determinators of low back pain. When in shape, the shapely waist curve is elliptical, like that of a racetrack. When your dietary consumption involves many irresistible extra scoops and when your daily exercise regimen is merely a hoot, the sexy human ellipsoid transforms itself into the human hoola hoop...it's circular and makes noises when jiggling from the hips. This very visual anatomical evidence of a hoola hoop-shaped waistline is to be given serious consideration when looking for determinators of low back pain. The hoola hoop determinator is a predominant condition amongst the North American population—predominant enough that this common hoola hoop human form will, one day, be identified as its own human medical breed: Humanus lardicus.

Humanus lardicus: a condition of the waistline, affecting only humans, that upsets the belly-to-back balance visually and mechanically, creating both sore eyes and sore mechanosis.

In construction, walls must have studs placed at equidistant intervals from each other. Cutting corners will increase the risk of crumbling corners! Our fleshy front, back, and side walls must also be strong to support a heavy and active upper body. Contracted abdominal walls, strong lumbar erectors, and sidewall muscles are the key structures to avoid a hell of a human hoola hoopin' mechanosis back problem. Being strong all around and avoiding the growth of an astronomical orbital ring around "planet waist" will, we all know, eliminate the human hoola hoop determinator.

6. THE DEGENERATE DETERMINATOR...NOT BETTER LATE THAN NEVER

Warning! This section contains a subject matter of a mature nature. Some may find it offensive. Others may see it as eye-opening. Those with weak stomachs and fragile egos need not read beyond the first paragraph of this section. Knowing the title of this section will be sufficient, stating simply that "degeneration" is a determinator factor. If you choose to read beyond this point, you will be reading at your own risk and discretion. The subject matter shared in this section is very much the opinion of the writer. It contains graphic scenes of unattractive bare boned nudity.

RAINY RIMADYL MORNINGS

Reading the pharmaceutical ad in my monthly fitness mag (as cheap a motivating personal trainer as they come) it became clear to me how people don't think of themselves as equal and vulnerable degenerating candidates to their dogs.

Rimadyl, a pharmaceutical product that controls the inflammation component of arthritis, is marketed using the resultant effects of a dog's arthritis on the owner's lifestyle. These marketing geniuses ask you to answer questions about your dog. The scene depicts a little girl sitting at the top of the stairs looking down on her Golden Lab, whose chin is resting on the first step. She's still holding onto his leash. Don't let your dog's arthritis come between you and him. The ad asks you to consider the following:

1. Does your dog tire easily after long walks?
2. Does your dog limp, lag behind, or appear stiff after activity?

3. Is your dog reluctant to climb stairs or jump up?

4. Is your dog slow to rise from a resting position?

If you answered yes to any of these questions, your dog may have arthritis, or even worse, you may have dog-arthritis! Believe me when I say that I know what you're thinking about right now. That's why I've begun the Degenerate Determinator section with an awakening dose of Rimadyl. Four out of four, you have probably answered yes...not for your dog, but for yourself, right? "Get me some Rimadyl with my morning coffee, please."

SOONER OR LATER

The inevitable will arrive, and the later the better! The Degenerative Determinator will arrive, but that doesn't mean it should force you into an early confinement to a walker. When your vertebral count has superseded your dental count, you can be sure the years of spinal wearing are a contributing low back pain determinator.

With the slow going of weakening human tissues, in combination with the progressive destructive effects of chronic disorderly mechanosis, we age. These inner weakenings are progressive, just like the creeping lil' dermal depressions developing in the corners of your eyes from the years of mechanosis action of your shining smiles. How much longer can we hide behind the makeup and magical airbrush?

Is time the enemy? Fact is, time itself wears us out. The ticking of time takes its toll on our biological clock. As we move along from rust to dust, with time, cartilage, ligaments, and the surrounding spinal tissues begin showing their age.

As time goes by, it ages us. Time attacks disc tissues, eventually drying them up like an old abandoned dish sponge. Time ruins everything and everything eventually tries to ruin your flexibility. Aged bones attempt to link to one another with spurs. These spurs act like a helping hand that is reaching out to grab your own outstretched hand that is attached to your cliff-hanging body. It is usually yesteryears of mechanosis disorders that will cause a weakening and breakdown of spinal tissues. Time becomes the enemy. You solidify, and then petrify. Your body soon takes on the personality of a white hair: it's stiff, it's coarse, it doesn't bend very well, and it sticks out. Frightening, isn't it?

RAIN PAIN

If you can even delay for one year the inevitable meteorological psychic gift you will one day receive (Boy, do I feel bad weather coming on!), is it not worth your efforts to stick to the program that may just delay the inevitable for as long as you can? Would you not stick with a program saving you from progressive degeneration with an eye-opening view on how to delay and lessen that frightening degenerate determinator? The other option is clear: to continue with your blind living plan and be the first to show just how much you have reaped what your life has sown. "Poor old man, he can hardly walk—he must have been a bricklayer in his old country."

THE JURASSIC SPINAL EPIDEMIOLOGIST

Radiological historians will be able to tell you what kind of life you had in your yesteryears. Your lumbar numbers four (L4) and five (L5) will very likely be the levels hit first, showing up like male pattern balding and receding hairline, as thinning and shrinking discs, growing spurs, and dwindling body height. I'll put a hundred on L5 first, please! It'll be the first to go. It's where, mechanically speaking, most of life's punches hit first.

Today's "40s and up" club members were hit with hard times in their youth—hit by hard gravity forces, intensified by sporting flat canvas runners (pre-Nike world) used in gym class, and camel hair mats (before sponge mats) to help brace our gymnastic falls. One day, the spinal epidemiologist will be able to show his colleague archaeologists all the signs found in our millennium-aged spinal bones that show just how hard we worked to create the "anti-germicidal", digital, and "pro-industrial" world we live in today. Spines don't lie! They show the evidence of degeneration as a result of the unfortunate "No-World" we used to live in: no dishwasher, no lightweight irons, no washer and dryer, no vacuum cleaner, no polisher, no tractor, no plow, no backhoe, no forklift. It will be an archaeology student who will one day give a name to the discovery of a mass of old human bones amongst the ruins of our Millennium civilization: "Professor, come see what I have discovered. What do you think these were?" The professor answers the question: "I believe this site was once an orthopedic hospital site. These look like the bones of a species called the 'Spinasorass'." He continues to help his student understand: "The Spinasorass suffered a great deal during this evolutionary period called the 'No-World.'" They sure did!

Today, we send our thanks to Home Depot for bringing Black and Decker and Dewalt into our lives to help lessen gravity's effects on our aging bones. The forces of nature on our spines have been lessened with the advancement of the industrial movement.

SPINAL SCARS AND SPINAL SCARES: WHAT DO YOU THINK?

At what age, do you think, is the point of no return—the point where signs of spinal decay begin to show on x-ray? Believe it or not, we're all grown up by the time we reach twenty, and we can't hide the evidence, either. The very first stages of arthritis (osteo-arthritis, degenerative disc disease, for example) can be present in the old bones of a young twenty year old—a stage identified by altered bone positions...positions out of position!

Conservative views on the definition of degeneration call it a downsizing phenomenon. Medical school's popular Dorland's Medical Dictionary describes it as "a change from a higher to a lower form, especially change of tissue to a lower or less functionally active form." A subentry to this definition needs to be added. It is a determinator factor, not yet discussed, that is a cause of degeneration. It is a determinator factor that indirectly causes low back pain, and should therefore be added to the list of determinators. The definition's subscript should read: degeneration is the consequence of our unaccountable neglect!

8

THE GUILTY TRIAD

It is my belief that there are three determinators of back pain that my Sexy Back program can repair, fix and even cure. Low back pain determinators are weak abdominals: people get the back bends from poorly supported, bulging, flabby tummies. Another common determinator is lack of flexibility. However, in my opinion, the number one reason why people get low back pain originates from the flat-as-a-pancake, shapeless North American ass!

The Flat Ass family is a popular one. The "spinaflatass tribe" is everywhere. All flattery aside, it is very connected to other contributing causes like bony alignment problems, alordotic bony positions, amorphous bony art, asymmetric bony arrangement, and atrophic lumbar muscles.

The real truth about why most of us get back pain has been revealed and it is not as complicated as you might think. Your pain is caused by the shortcomings of agility, ass, and abdominals. For some, the truth about what's causing their back pain may be awfully hard to face. Today's bad back is a unique plague characterized by distinct anatomical originalities and abnormalities. I call these three physical blips "The Guilty Triad." The Guilty Triad is inarguably connected to our so very comfy and so very e-equipped times. The Guilty Triad is enabled by carelessness and ignorance and is inarguably a precipitator of our very own biological destruction! Who would have guessed that through its own creepy and sneaky insertion into our lives, The Guilty Triad has such a powerful negative force beyond mere physical degradation?

Be aware and do not downplay the terrible power of The Guilty Triad. You have likely been ignoring the presence of these typical determinator factors for years now. The Guilty Triad is a major contributor to the back pain plague of our times. Pay attention and be on the watch for the more fashionable and universal determinators of low back pain I call The Guilty Triad: the blubbery bellies or weakened abs, the collapsed buttery butts of a flat ass, and the lack of agility cause by unbending muscles tightly binding your bones!

The agility, abdominal and ass factors stand firmly behind the "mechano", "myo", "inflammo", "neuro", and "arthro" categorical pathologies. They are the all-too-important faults that contribute immensely to these five categories of back pathologies.

THE PROOF OF THE GUILTY TRIAD

Medicine demonstrates the validity of its new therapeutic discoveries in three ways: with quantified studies, with controlled studies and with anatomical analysis. Essentially, we test thousands in quantified studies and if thousands of others got the same results, then it must work. Or in controlled studies we only give the treatment to half of the guinea pigs and we pretend to medicate the other half and see what happens. Then, the geniuses at oDesk figure it all out for you...were the differences conclusively significant or not? Or we take things apart to see if we changed things around in there.

So let's test our theory. The Shopping Network has already tested and shown the evidence that back strain has a direct connection to the blubbery belly (thank you Dr. Ho), so only the importance of the agility and ass factors in The Guilty Triad equation needs to be proven. The making of a bad back can be demonstrated with a simple maneuver: Lie on the floor and then get up. Getting back on your feet will require the cooperation of all three parts of The Guilty Triad. The task of lifting yourself off the floor not only requires a strong, intact abdominal wall; it also needs the combining support from the other two Triad components: an agile spine and a curvy ass. If you can't pick yourself up off the floor, you can pretty much count on having one of The Guilty Triad components missing in your life.

First, lie on your back, knees bent, ankles touching butt (as close to your buttocks as can be) and arms at your side. This is your starting point. (Refer to position 1) The end position is not raising yourself completely up on your feet, but raising yourself up to the torso-to-thigh contact (see Proof Test Test 1) point. Getting up to a torso-to-thigh contact demonstrates full ability of your abs, your curvy ass and your agility.

You can try to complete this maneuver in three different ways: One is super easy, one is very difficult, and one is a middle ground called "the neutral point." The neutral point is the one that can be used as a comparison of what feels easier or what feels more difficult. It will test the middle point between a disadvantaged spine and an advantaged one, and it will help determine just how independent and important each component of The Guilty Triad is.

From the "ready for take-off" position, similar to the starting position for a sit-up, lift your torso up and aim for torso-to-thigh contact. No need to hold the position. No need to strain yourself. No matter how high you were able to reach, you will use this feeling and height as the measure to compare your strength with the next two moves.

The next test is performed with Agility being compromised, followed by the third test using an overly exaggerated Ass.. Theoretically, with one factor missing (Agility), one can assume that the outcome will be a task that is more difficult to perform. When adding an excess of another component, this test will be easier to perform. One must keep in mind that the Abs component of The Guilty Triad is involved in all three tests. Agility is tested in the second maneuver and Ass in the third the baseline is a true measure of your Abs' contribution in the act of lifting yourself off to get to your knees. Ready for your second launch?

THE PROOF TEST

TEST 1

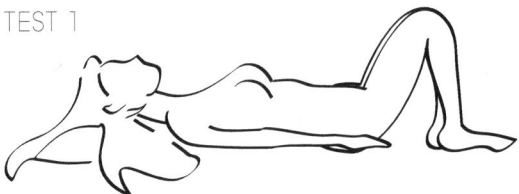

Lie on your back, knees bent, ankles touching butt (as close to your buttocks as can be) and arms at your side. This is your starting point.

TEST 2

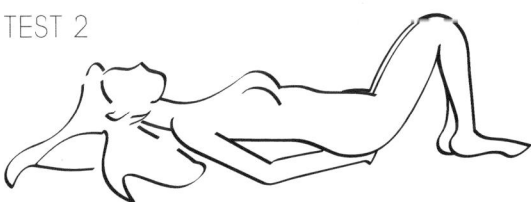

To remove Agility, make fists with both hands, and then place them underneath your tush. This position locks the lumbar vertebras in a flexed and therefore immobile position.

TEST 3

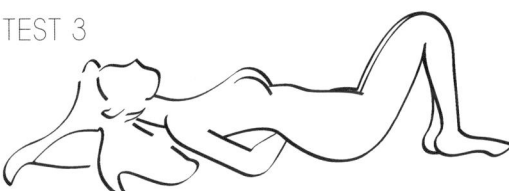

Place your hands above your tush. When looking from the side, your low back curve is smoothly rounded, making your ass look perfect.

In this same position, the importance of Agility is demonstrated by removing it from your back while trying to get to completion (see Proof Test, Test 2). The idea is to make you miss Agility once it's gone. To remove Agility, make fists with both hands, and then place them underneath your tush. Fists squished by your behind, the pelvis is lifted up from the ground. This position locks the lumbar vertebras in a flexed and therefore immobile position. This is one way to remove the Agility factor in The Guilty Triad. When the vertebras are in a flexed position, they are more difficult to move.

To further illustrate the "agility and flexing" concept, try looking to the right with your neck while keeping your head well-positioned over your shoulders. Then try again, this time with your chin tucked in and head all the way down before trying to look to the right. It's much more difficult to rotate when in a flexed position. This experiment works on any joint with flexing capabilities. Try it with your finger, rotating (twisting) it passively in a straight position, and then try to do the right and left finger twisting rotation again with your finger completely extending back. Ouch!

With your squished fists under your tush, the resulting flexed pelvis and lumbar spine position means you have lost a big part of your free inter-segmental (one vertebra on top of the other) movement. There is no flexibility in your lower back, so our maneuver will be done with Agility removed from the equation. Remember that this is an experiment by way of comparison. Rise with no hands under buttock. Rise with hands under buttock. Is there a difference? Power to Agility! Power to lumbar flexibility! And now, remove your fist before you lose all the power to your fingers.

For the next test you will feel the power difference when you try to get to the finish line without an Ass (see Proof Test, Test 3). Remember that when discussing the Ass component of The Guilty Triad, we're discussing the importance of a lordosis in your low back. Lordosis, the normal dipping curve your lumbar bones make when aligned properly, is the normal anatomical position of your lower backbones. When taken away, the alordotic position makes your back and ass unattractively look shapeless and flattened. No lordosis—no ass because the flattened lumbar line goes right down to your ass, making it look flat. The sexy gluteal curves of your butt disappear when you lose the curve of your low back.

Going back to our experiment, in the neutral position (hands at your side), when trying to get to the finishing torso-to-thigh position, your low back was already flattened to the ground. By way of comparison, let your hands do the magic by placing them above your derriere, into the hollow of your back, to create the normal lordotic curve. Another option is to place a rolled towel in the hallow of your back.When looking from the side, your low back curve is smoothly rounded, making your ass look perfect. Hands in their lumbar place, filling the space between the floor and your curved back, try to get up to the finish line without using your hands or arms to push yourself up from the ground. With record speed, I bet, this was a breeze. By giving you your lordosis back, comparing it to the flattened position, the difference is instantly seen and felt.

Agility, Abdominals, and Ass: the three A's of The Guilty Triad team. When investigating why people develop back pain, one should start by looking into my concept called The Guilty Triad for the answers. Strong enough to create dysfunction when present alone, they almost always present themselves as a bunch of co-dependent back buddies. So how do we fix our pain problem?

9

THE BIG FIX:
THE TORSO THREESOME

Remember The Sisy Squat Sex Test? Well, it's baaaaack! The Sisy Squat Sex Test is also the all-encompassing Torso Threesome tester. To perform with ease and success you need the best of balance between the three concepts I have called Torso Curve, Torso Rhythm, and Torso Hoop. Missing any of the three will make The Sex Test impossible to pass. A good test score means a good balance between the three torsos; and a good balance between the Sexy Back's threesome means a hot performer when it comes to twosome action.

The theory of Occam's razor is that all things being equal, the simplest explanation will be the right one. For scientists this theory applies when the inquisitive mind is tossing between two competing theories that make exactly the same predictions. With this in mind, I have assembled some simple solutions to heal back pain while solving The Guilty Triad's three A's (Ass, Agility and Abs) with reparative solutions I call The Torso Threesome: Torso Rhythm, Torso Curves and Torso Hoop.

THE TORSO THREESOME NUMBER ONE: TORSO RHYTHM

Immobility kills! Move it, or lose it. With the millions of expressive facial images, billions of body language poses, trillions of living movements, and gazillions of combinations between those millions, billions, and trillions of possibilities, we move and show the world every moment of the day our moving individualities.

With immobility comes fusion: fusion of your bones and fusion of your world. Torso Rhythm defies fusion. Keeping our torsos moving keeps things loose, feeds stiff joints with a fresh splash of synovial fluids. Torso rhythm keeps your mechanical innards warm and supple, circulating and purifying your body fluids, and soaking and lubricating your tissue fluids.

THE TORSO THREESOME NUMBER TWO: TORSO CURVE

Torso Curve, the second component of the Torso Threesome, refers to a dynamic lordosis. Our natural curves are as aero-dynamic as an airplane's wing to make us fly high through both the heaviness of life's whirlwinds and the heavy loads of life's luggage! A lordotic low back curve defines the Torso Curve component of The Torso Threesome.

We have poorly designed innards when it comes to sitting. You already know that! Yet, other than a good sofa, which ranks as second best spot in the world to relax, it also is definitely our most frequently used position in the world. Our genetic spinal manufacturer has given us very limited warranties. It makes sense that a working spine suffers less in the long run when compared to a long sitting one. Sitting is a negative power force on our bony frames.

Torso Curve will help reduce the back beatings of a sitting spine. The lumbar lordosis will anatomically reposition everything where it belongs, which will minimize the physical weight-bearing forces of the upper body on the lumbar spine. With Torso Curve, low back disc pressure is minimal and with cooperation from Torso Curve, the sitting pelvic position is safer.

To demonstrate further the importance of Torso Curve, remember that with Torso Curve preserved you can withstand five to eight thousand Newton units of pressure on your back. For those whose forte does not include physics, eight thousand Newton means that it is less than the weight of a car but more that of than an upright piano. What part of the body gives way beyond the weight of eight Newton? The bones! Discs are stronger than bone when Torso Curve is preserved. When Torso Curve is removed it is the posterior part of the disc (closest to the central canal that houses your spinal cord, AKA boy star part number seven, Chapter 3) that gives way. Without Torso Curve, discs collapse. Sitting removes Torso Curve. Sitting, therefore, affects discs first. It doubles the pressure on the discs when compared to standing.*

*Some Really Technical Info: Where does all the action occur? Your x-rays will show it, your brain will feel it, and the academics to follow will confirm it. When turning Torso Curve into torso "alordosis," where does all the disc pressure go? Most of the movement happens at the bottom level, lumbar number five (L5). When bending forward and backwards, most is at L5 (20 degrees) and decreases as you go up (12 degrees) at L1. In bending side-to-side, most is at L5, too (36 degrees), and decreases as you go up (6 degrees at L1). In rotation twists, most is at L5 (5 degrees), and decreases as you go up (2 degrees at L1). Your L5 is the most popular and active one of the bunches, meaning that when under stress, anything that causes you to lose your Torso Curve, L5 will most likely be the one to be hit first. It makes sense, at this point, to say that restoring Torso Curve is the best way to cool down all the heat created down there.

THE TORSO THREESOME NUMBER THREE: TORSO HOOP

An army is only as strong as its weakest soldier. Likewise, your back is only as strong as its weakest vertebral complex. Your back is made up of a whole gang of human tissue teammates who need each other's support to make a strong, effective back team. Your back troop is a big part of the Torso Hoop.

If you trace the contours of your waistline, palpating front, sides, and back, you'll see that you need the entire hoop's cooperation for back strength and function. The troop is made up of three team members: your back, composed of bones, discs, muscles, and all their holding elements; your side muscle wall; and—surprise, surprise—your front abdominal wall, whether it's buried—or not—by a coat of adipose tissue (fat).

BLACK BACK BELT

Maximizing Torso Hoop with the use of a back belt support is a long debated subject when weighing its efficacy and validity. Perhaps the decision should be left in the hands of the suffering back patient. A quick fitting session in the back of your nearest medical or fitness supply store will help give you the personal experience to measure its effect on your own suffering back. You can decide for yourself if there is an empowering difference for you.

The Late Joe Weider, Ironman Father, has always been a firm (and well-muscled) backer of the "yea" supporters of back belts for back power. His wife, Betty, is the world's most beautiful role model (37–18–36) and spokesperson for the use of back belts amongst women during weight lifting exercises. Betty's Torso Hoop beauty speaks louder than any medical words. No doubt she does not suffer from any spinal ills.

There are other belt benefits that generate a "yea" interest in bodybuilding. The belt assists in physically pushing your backbones into a Torso Curved lordotic position. It also provides psychological feedback, reminding its wearer to "think back safety"!

INSPECTOR GADGET

The magic behind getting sexy six-pack abs does not come from the doings of one particular exercise. If this were true your Shopping Network browsing time would significantly be reduced. After you've decided on which Shopping Network personal gadget will work best for you—or which model you want to look like the most—your consistent efforts in working those abs (200 crunches a day keeps Torso Hoop alive and back pain away) is only one part of Jillian Michaels, Shaun T and Tony Horton's promises. Take note that Torso Hoop can only be effective if abdominal wall contractions are sustained. How then, do you think, those Baywatch washboards stay ripped for the entire hour? Keeping the abdominals contracted at all times is how Torso Hoop is kept alive.

STUPID HUMAN TRICKS

David Letterman, who introduced the world to Stupid Human Tricks, consistently does a stupid human trick of his own as his way of warming up the audience at the start of his Late Night shows. With straight locked legs he bends over and touches his toes. "Look Ma, no Torso Curve, and at that bent-over angle, no Torso Hoop either." Let's just hope that he will have an eternity of Torso Rhythm power to get him back up to face his audience. Bending over without bending at the knees is old fashioned, downright dangerous, and frankly, the very best—or worst—of stupid human tricks. Maybe Mr. Letterman should skip the Stupid Human Trick and play with his funny bones instead. He should get on the floor to do his "smart human trick" by picking one of the four solo sexercises you're about to learn.

MAKING THE BACK-SEX CONNECTION

How then, are Torso Rhythm, Torso Curve, and Torso Hoop connected to sex, and how are they used as a cure to the single suffering spine? Having lost your Agility, Abs, and Ass curves may be a literal bummer, but discovering that the loss of these three anatomical concepts is connected to your back pain may have awakened a new understanding within you. Identifying, defining, and understanding The Torso Threesome will help all those interested in the active self-help approach to fixing back pain. Letting your Agility, Abs, or Ass deteriorate will make you susceptible to suffering. Self-preservation of a well working Torso Threesome is how you avoid a breakdown of The Guilty Triad.

Each component of the Torso Threesome touches upon the rumba action in partnered sexual passion. Learning how each torso component is connected with your moves of passion is exactly how you will understand and, if you're lucky, get to the peaks of your sexual passion to help fix your, or someone else's, lumbar malfunctions.

SKEW-ME

The sex and spine connection was awakened in my head by the many early Monday morning chats I had with patients. Sex, as healer of the bad back, came to mind when my chronically suffering female patients came boasting they had just had more than a lucky weekend of serious climactic pleasures. The women were eager to tell me that their back pain seemed to have gone into spontaneous remission after a weekend of sexual fixings. How could I not put two-and-two-and-too together? Two people, two days, and too good to be true! Any physician would have had to be closed-minded and clinically blind to miss this connection! Since sexual history is not on the doctor's list of first-visit questions to ask a patient with back pain, the connection between back pain and sex was truly an unbiased discovery.

Suddenly, I—pain relieving doctor—am obsolete. All back pain is cured with a prescription of safe sex three times a week. When prescribing sex as medicine for your back pain, the side effects and warning signs of an overdose should read: If taken in excess the patient may experience feelings of euphoria, ecstasy, rapture, and bliss.

THE COMING AROUND OF YOUR CYCLE OF LIFE

Sex touches upon the three torso solutions in eliminating low back pain. The average doctor will weigh many common benefits to sexual pleasures other than, well, pleasures. In my opinion I choose to put pleasure at the very top of the list. Right behind "low back power"! Sex for pleasure is good for you!

Sex is a fat burner. Do it three times a week for a modest burning of 7,500 calories a year; the equivalent of running 75 miles a year. Show me a person who would prefer to pound the pavement for the same caloric loss and I'll show you a back pain sufferer who should be pounding his head on the pavement instead. When a 170-pound person fools around for 50 minutes, 90 calories will have been burned.

Sex leads to healthier, lustier living and release of tension. The French call the big "O" La Petite Mort, meaning "The

Little Death." This climactic metaphor means it is the little death of your internal misery. It is the little death of your bottled-up tension. Sex aids your body's chemicals. It helps lower cholesterol and brings the good fats (the high-density lipoprotein—HDL) into balance. Sex activates your cardio-respiratory system. Blood turns rich red and breath rate becomes deeper and faster. Sex releases endorphins (your brain's natural reserve of morphine) to numb your painful knots, nerves, muscles, and bones. It raises testosterone levels in men. It is believed that raised testosterone and endorphins are natural analgesics, acting like anti-inflammatories. Sounds like N. Erv Stension, Sue Wellings, and Art Wrightess should be having MMW a threesome.

For men sex is the only activity that helps flush the prostate. A recent British Medical Journal (B.M.J. is synonymous with truth and respect) study has shown that five to seven weekly sex sessions can extend a man's life. The studs studied were shown to have 50% lower risk of death than their abstinent counterparts.

It has been shown that DHEA (Dehydroepiandrosterone, a naturally occurring hormone) spikes three to five times its normal serum concentration just before your own spiking climax. DHEA has been talked up for being an immune system booster, tumor growth inhibitor, and bone growth promoter. I'd settle for helping with just a bit of home-improvement handy-man skills myself.

Saving the sexy best for last is...you will look like and feel like a Betta Luva! You will instantly look better. You will glow like you just lost ten pounds. You will stand taller, think more positively, be a knockout in bed, and become a good consumer of potential sex partners. And if your mother has always sworn that you had a healing gift, then this is as good a reason as any to reach out and touch someone!!!

Sex is exercise, and with exercise comes another list of benefits. And just so you understand that my exercises aren't homework, I've given them an appropriate name. The cornerstone of my program is sexercise: the combination of exercise and sex for the double-tasking benefit of personal and spinal wellness. If that's not motivation, then what is?

10

THE WHAM BAM PROGRAM—YOUR PLACE OR MINE?

Looking back, it was a difficult task sifting through the never-ending list of so-called "helpful prescriptive exercises" (you know, the ones you were never really going to do anyway, even when weighed down by the worst of kinked and locked-up back bones) and selecting the most effective and uncomplicated ones. Even more difficult was to match effectively the crippling diagnostic realities (like self-induced forces called The Guilty Triad) with an easy-fit and quick-fix methodology. In the making of a new back-healing magic, I threw away the conventional and the boring, but well-intentioned, historic "same-old" solutions. Out with the ordinary and in with the extraordinary formula! A new science had to be invented to create a newfound love for spine science. A science that would change your faith!

I knew that if I could come up with a sexy science that would use love in the making of a strong back, then I had higher odds for success.

As difficult as it was cracking down on the long list of exercise finalists for the program, it was a breeze when compared to screening all the sexual position possibilities. Da Vinci could not have, in his entire lifetime, scribbled, chiseled, and chipped away all of the touching twosome possibilities himself. Too many possibilities, and thank goodness for that! Evaluating, eliminating, and re-inventing solo exercises was more than doubly complicated when it came to examining the diversity of duo contact! So many positions, so many pleasures, and so little time to enjoy those pleasures!

In the process of selecting that perfect pack, I realized that setting too many sex rules was not the way to go. Let's not forget that the task was to fabricate a Sexy Back program that would be lovingly uncomplicated. In the mass confusion of deciphering, assessing, picking, dissecting, and sometimes, even trying out what was available, the biggest reality check was the realization that the connection between the broken back and sex has always been there... long before man stopped sporting Neanderthal loincloth. I know you thought I invented sex, spines, and the best sex test pickup line in the world. Well, I will take credit for The Sisy Squat Sex Test pickup line and the techniques of my sexercises, but as far as sex and spines are concerned, my contribution was only to put in print what always was and should have been a long time ago! In the invention of a back-fixing sex program, my work simply involved the task of shaking your awareness with a few tricks that teach you a way to fix your back or someone else's with either solo or duo action.

REALITY BITES

Avocados, tomatoes, grapes, and testicles—a wicker basket with things that are spherical, things that are painfully squishable, and things that are not edible if blue! But one of these things doesn't belong with the others. Which one of these things doesn't belong with the others? Can you pick out the oddball in this basket? On the assumption that the tomatoes are green, you probably selected the male spheroids as the oddballs. Perhaps you should have selected a fruit ball instead. Why? Because you can't fool the medics! Come on now, we know you don't eat half the fruits you should be eating, which makes avocados, tomatoes, and grapes the oddball things in the basket sitting on your lap.

On the assumption that your present exercise regimen is as complete as your daily fruit intake, I have eliminated the unnecessary and re-invented the get-real, time-no-longer-wasted back exercise program. Knowing that your present exercise regimen is very likely as complete and commit-ted as your eight to twelve daily fruit servings, I want to make sure that the bites you do take will be the right ones. Think of Sexy Back as therapy for the "fruitophobics" and "fitnophobics" that we really are. Now that's not hard to swallow, is it? After all…eight to twelve fruits and veggies a day? We've got to be kidding, right?

And so, having interviewed just about every bartender south of 42nd and fast-forwarded my way through every adult flick I could find, I was able to keep myself sober, out of trouble, and focused on picking the best out there—not best adult video, best support bra, or best bartending advice, either—just best exercise and best sex moves for Sexy Back. Now we have the launch of a gifted program for all the lads and ladies who are single, suffering, and downright lazy. It was grueling research and exhausting punishment, but someone had to do it.

THE GIFTED PROGRAM: PARTS I AND II

For those who go-go solo, for those who are more spectators in the game of life, for those who prefer to scratch their own backs, for those who think of themselves as lone strangers, for those who turn away the helping hand, for those who prefer to be single handed, for those who would sooner savor the smell of magazine perfume strips on the pillow next to theirs, and finally, for those who guiltlessly prefer to give themselves a hand, there exists a practicum—a solo simulation program designed to accommodate the independent ones who prefer not to open a joint account with anyone. If this is you, then I welcome you to In Vitro: the practicum of Sexy Back. This part of the program involves solo sexercises: exercises designed to replace duo sexing action.

For those into body parts, for those who want to share, and for those who think solo only when they really have to, there exists a practical part to Sexy Back. I welcome you to In

Vivo! It is the opposite of In Vitro, involving lots of loving and "sexing." Sexing: the performance of selected sexercise movements in the company of a sex partner.

In Vitro is divided into two subsections, categorized according to their experimental environments: public and private. The public and private subsections each contain two sexercises. The two public sexercises are deemed appropriate to perform in the public eye of your local park, lunchroom, or gym. The two private sexercises are designed for the privacy of your home. All four sexercises have different names. All are performed in sets and repetitions (reps). In Sexy Back talk, sets are called "multiples" and reps are called "humps." The sexercises are performed in two multiples of ten humps for a total of twenty humps. All sexercises (and sexing moves, too!) finish with the same stretch break. Each sexercise takes less than one minute to perform, which means that you can easily squeeze in a couple of quickies in less than two minutes if you want to! And so I ask you, how hard can that be?

The first sexercise of each subsection is the more powerful yet, lucky for the lazy spazzed-out herds out there, the more passive. The second sexercise of each subsection is designed for strength, turning your resting vitals into heart throbbing, muscle twitching, heavy breathing, vocal grunting, and dermal dripping action...they're hot and they're sexy! You will never be asked to perform more than one subsection at a time. Each is to be performed either twice a day, after long sitting periods, or anytime as a low back pain reliever. The second active part of each sexercise subsection is optional. Performing this once every other day will suffice. Lots of options—lots of love!

ENOUGH IS ENOUGH?

Is that it? Is that all there is to the In Vitro part of the program? Is this really enough? Is a two-sexercise passive-active plan a good trade-off for back pain relief? Hold the questions and first ask yourself this: if more were given, would I be inclined to do them all? Even if you knew that with ten hours of hot sexing action three times a week for one month you would be promised ten pounds off, you still probably wouldn't get involved. But if you have time to tweeze, cut, clip, wax, shave, trim, pick and pull, then you can find time to hump, too! Besides, both beautician bodywork and Sexy Back pluck away at our physical vanity, don't they? With just two sexercises at hand (remember that you are only required to perform either one of two public or one of two private sexercises), and with only a few house rules tagging along with them, then just maybe new hope can be put back into the single back. You think? I hope!

With only two sexercises to perform, the program can hardly be called "another time-sucking addiction to add to your list." An addiction is the last thing any of us need to add to our lives. Living in "no-time" land, a time-deprived society where toothpaste tube flip-caps prevail over the screw-on type, where hisses are heard over our shoulders should we decide to do more than just a cash withdrawal transaction at the bank machine, where we can't be bothered to add that extra can of water to complete the canned soup recipe, where we'd slap any patch on our asses to quick-fix just about anything, who wants a new time-sucking addiction, anyway?

Are the program's four sexercises really enough? The short answer is yes! But to justify my righteousness, the program can only be "enough" if it forgives The Guilty Triad: no Agility, no Ass, and no Abs.

To make a perfect choice, I created fifteen sexercises and chose the ones that had the therapeutic properties necessary to fix our three inherent North American spinal sore spots: Agility, Ass, and Abs. And with all the sexercising for solo action and sexing for duo action torso intertwinements at play, the only way the program could have therapeutic benefit was to make sure these sexercises and sexing moves touched upon The Terrific Threesome. Otherwise, why waste even a minute with In Vitro sexercising or In Vivo sexing? Torso sexercises and sexing moves that involve Curve, Rhythm, and Hoop are the therapeutic powers used to solve the bad back attacks from the failures of Agility, Ass, and Abs!

SUCKING ON TIME

Most exercise programs have exhausting lists of time-sucking exercises. However, for some people, when actually trying some of them, you realize there's just the one. The one important one that holds all the healing powers on its shoulders—the one that just seems to loosen you up—the one that makes you feel more limber—the one that seems to give you the most pain relief—and the one that makes you last longer...and as for the other ones… In Vitro is just that: "The One!" It's the healing one. It is the one important move that actually holds all the power in the exercise program. The other ones, well, are simply runners-up.

DISCLAIMING DOCTRINAIRE DISCLAIMERS?

Before embarking on In Vitro sexercises or In Vivo sexing, are there any limits you should know about? Limits that, if not respected, would take you into deeper suffering? Are there Surgeon General warnings that you should know about? Should you be afraid when approaching your own crybaby pain threshold limits? Is it possible to obtain gains without pains? Should you be looking for a sign saying you must be at least thirty-six inches tall to ride this goose bump, "coif"—raising program? Are you looking for the warning sign above your ass that says "keep-out—trespassers will be prosecuted"?

As far as Sexy Back is concerned, rather than looking for just about any reason not to participate, perhaps you should be looking for the more important sign that's pointing to your head, not your ass. A sign that reads: "Use Your Head Instead!" And if after you've tried using your head you still find yourself questionably empty-headed and paranoid as hell about participating in this program from the fear of even bigger back bumps and bruises, then consult not the physician, not the nurse, and not the paralegal, either. Seek the help of a local community center's accredited fitness professional—one who will understand when it's time to begin and when it's time to stop! But most of all, try to rely on and confidently trust your head to tell you if something doesn't feel right down there. Remember that simplicity is the key to enjoy-ability. Remember that sensitivity and sensibility are the incoming brain messages to look for in order to avoid dis-ability. And finally, remember that sensuality is where it's at to restore "move-ability" and "sex-ability." Take responsibility for your life and enjoy it.

On your behalf, dozens of existing workout programs and hundreds of exercises have been screened and executed, and a selected powerful four sexercises were either modified or re-invented. The program has been set up to work for you. And for those eager to embark on the In Vivo sexing program, it is still crucial that all In Vivo participants learn the In Vitro moves first. In Vitro will prepare you well for In Vivo sessions. In Vitro practice will increase the therapeutic efficacy of In Vivo moves. You don't want to be stepping on anyone's toes, elbowing someone in the mouth, or resting elbows on someone's hair when playing ménage-a-deux. Starting the program lessons with the In Vitro section is a requirement. If you commit, then soon you will be replacing all the emptiness underneath you with that special In Vivo filler you've been waiting for.

The In Vitro and In Vivo methods are programs. The power of In Vitro comes from the one source: specific physical movements that you will soon learn. Those movements are the physical driving forces of In Vitro. They are the power engines that drive your front end with maximum horsepower. To drive your front end, you need a good motor behind you.

The power of In Vivo, on the other hand, stems from three sources. The first is the same as In Vitro. The second is the long list of physical benefits you get from stress relief, calorie burning and getting more love. The third is the eye-opener that will change the way you think when you share your love: the exchange of a sexing physical energy that creates an interchange of soul energies. Chi, Feng Shui for the soul, is an interchanging occurrence. This exchange program feeds a large basis of In Vivo's "sexapeutic" effect—Sex Chi! Nothing granola and nothing Tantrum about that! Nothing to do with the Sigma Chi Titta fraternity, either! Just good vibes if you're sharing with the right one.

DISCOVER OSTEYOGA FOR THOSE LAZY BONES

Both In Vitro and In Vivo programs begin the same way. They both use the same concepts of curve, rhythm, and hoop—top three reasons to fix bottom three problems (Agility, Ass, and Abs). Both programs begin more passively (not "just-hit-me-again-please" sado-passive, but passive as in "just much less difficult"), and then progress to a more difficult, active level. If you never get to the second level, don't panic, because there will be no harm done. The power of the program is in the first part of In Vitro and In Vivo.

The second half is designed to build back strength, to make you stronger than ever, to make you (and it) last longer than ever, to make you look better than ever, and to give you more energy than ever! But for the pains, for the flexibility, for the pressure, for the reduction of recurrent strains, and let's not forget, for sexual vanity, then the passive part of In Vitro and In Vivo is downright good enough. The passivity of In Vitro and In Vivo's first part touches upon Torso Curve and Torso Rhythm. As discussed already the second, more active part involves all three parts of The Torso Threesome. Keeping with flexibility and movement is foremost on the "how to" list of sexy back fixings. The grueling hooping workouts can be performed "as an occasional only." Should you forfeit The Torso Hoop, just don't come crying on my medical table if you get beach sand kicked in your face this summer.

For the sake of your flattened ass curves and your dis-abilities to bend over all the way, do your "Osteyoga!" It's the word I've created to describe the moves you will do to loosen those bones of yours when alone...or not. Osteyoga is yoga for backbones. Osteyoga is for those who are bad to the bone. Osteyoga is purity—the safest, quickest, and most concentrated way to get you off the floor and off to more.

The Osteyoga exercises for the terrific Torso Threesome (Rhythm, Curve, and Hoop) are designed to fix The Guilty Triad (Agility, Ass, and Abs), which pretty much covers the majority of us. But remembering the many other less-popular determinators and categorical injury-types, more Osteyoga exercise moves may be needed.

In Vitro and In Vivo are designed to help all five categories of back problems. Remember that with The Guilty Triad problems comes the acquisition of different degrees of Stiffy, Puffy, Spazzy, Sparky and Creaky. And for some, the Stiffy, Puffy, Spazzy, Sparky, and Creaky categories of back problems may need more than In Vitro and In Vivo.

More severe disabling disorders and diseases can be found within these five determinator categories. Going beyond the In Vitro and In Vivo program should be considered if "the change" does not feel where you think it should be after one or two weeks into the program. Chances are high that if you're in it for your own back pain, then you can wait a couple of weeks to see if more is needed. But also remember that chances are that you won't! After a couple of weeks, the slightest of positive changes is a realistic and good sign that you're moving in the right direction. You should remember that sometimes the only way through the pain…is through the pain! We're not talking about your pain of origin here. What I mean is that feeling—the ache of exercise and body stiffness—is nothing to balk at when awakening positive healing changes within.

As you begin to learn the applications of In Vivo and In Vitro, you will need to learn the incoming spinal messages and judge for yourself what is deemed perfect, not enough effort, or too much. You will need to learn to feel what is therapeutic, what is under-treating or overdosing. Your best guide is to avoid "sharp" as the incoming brain message. Never ask yourself, "Is this normal pain?" Pain is not normal. If you feel a sharp pain during In Vitro or In Vivo, a familiar pain that is intense like the pain you want to get rid of in the first place, it will mean one of two things: A) Sorry, you are not a candidate for In Vitro or In Vivo because you fall into the "hot zone" acute back pain category. In Vitro and In Vivo are designed for chronic sufferers. If you are hot and acute (lots of sharpies back there), then that's a whole new chapter in itself—and I've called it "Love Hurts" (Chapter 13), or B) You are pushing yourself too much and the "sharp" message your brain is receiving is your back's way of saying "back it off a bit, will ya?! Your ranges of motion (how far you bend forward or backward) are too much at this time. It's okay to keep driving, but stay on the paved road and stop swaying beyond your own natural limits. Stick to what feels natural and what feels good!

So just what are you supposed to feel during your sexercising In Vitro or sexing In Vivo program? After all the "plié, relevé, developé" should you also expect "soufflii beaucoup"? Look not in the "feeling" for your answers as the answers lie in the "what not to feel." You don't want to feel anything "sharp," as in safety pin pricking, bee sting, thorn pricking, finger-in-door jamming, exposed molar nerve to a spoonful of ice cream, old wicker chair ass cheek pinching, nose hair plucking, and toe stubbing sharp. Your reflexes will tell you to avoid sharp pains. So what disclaimer do I have to assure In Vitro and In Vivo safety? Stay out of the sharp zone at all times, will ya?

Any change in a positive direction is good enough. Changes like reduction of pain intensity, reduction in the size of the pain area, improved spinal stamina, increased back range of motion, improved leg sensation, increased leg strength, and reduction of frequency of pain patterns are signs of excellent progress. If you feel you have reached a plateau after a couple of months, then perhaps, for some, given the pathology involved, that may be as good as it gets! As a realistic minimalist, only the essential is shared with you here. For most of us, this will be good enough. If I can get any suffering back to do at least this much, or if any physician can get a patient do at least two exercises on a regular basis, for that matter, then we should be thrilled, given that more than 75% of patients don't even finish taking their prescriptions.

For those wanting to jump into the In Vivo sack right away, be forewarned one last time that it is recommended that all suffering backs and sexicians in training begin with In Vitro first. The In Vitro Osteyoga program will help develop your In Vivo moves into therapy. Besides, in the absence of a duet partner, it's a good idea to learn how to play a good solo performance when you have to. And even in the presence of a duet partner, you never know when you will be asked to sleep on the couch!

IN VITRO: SEXERCISE IS MEDICINE

Time to go through the motions! Ready to learn what it takes to be a connoisseur of sexercise for back relief? First, you learn to lather, rinse, and repeat. That's right—Repeat! The instructions ask that you repeat after lathering and rinsing. But who's kidding who here? Who's got "repeat" time these days? How about just a one-time splatter, one-time rinse, and then flee? Personally, I have never had a shower with someone who took the time to lather twice. The only time I ever lather twice is in the morning, but only because I sometimes can't remember if I've lathered even once. The sexercise instruction in this back book is very much like a lather–rinse–repeat shampoo bottle, only if you don't have time for the "re's", you'll still come out smelling as sweet as chocolate almond scented massage oil.

The first of the two sexercises is the passive one. It can be performed by itself, as it holds its therapeutic weight quite well on its own. This first sexercise is an Osteyoga power move. The second sexercise is active, designed to re-strengthen the surrounding musculature to make you a stronger "liver" and a better lover. I am aware that you are being showered with repeating instructions but I would rather lather you up nicely now with these important instructions than see you throw in the towel later because you didn't read the instructions on the label right.

When in the public eye you will have a pair of sexercises that won't make you look like you're having a spontaneous passionate moment with your exercise mat. Those two sexercises are rated Adult Accompaniment, which means you can do them in the presence of others. So for me, rated (AA) means rated: X-posed.

I also have a different, yet similar, pair of sexercises presented for In Vivo prep's sake when you are alone, rated: X-rated. The X-rated sexercises are also split into a passive and active move. But remember these two sexercises are Rated X!

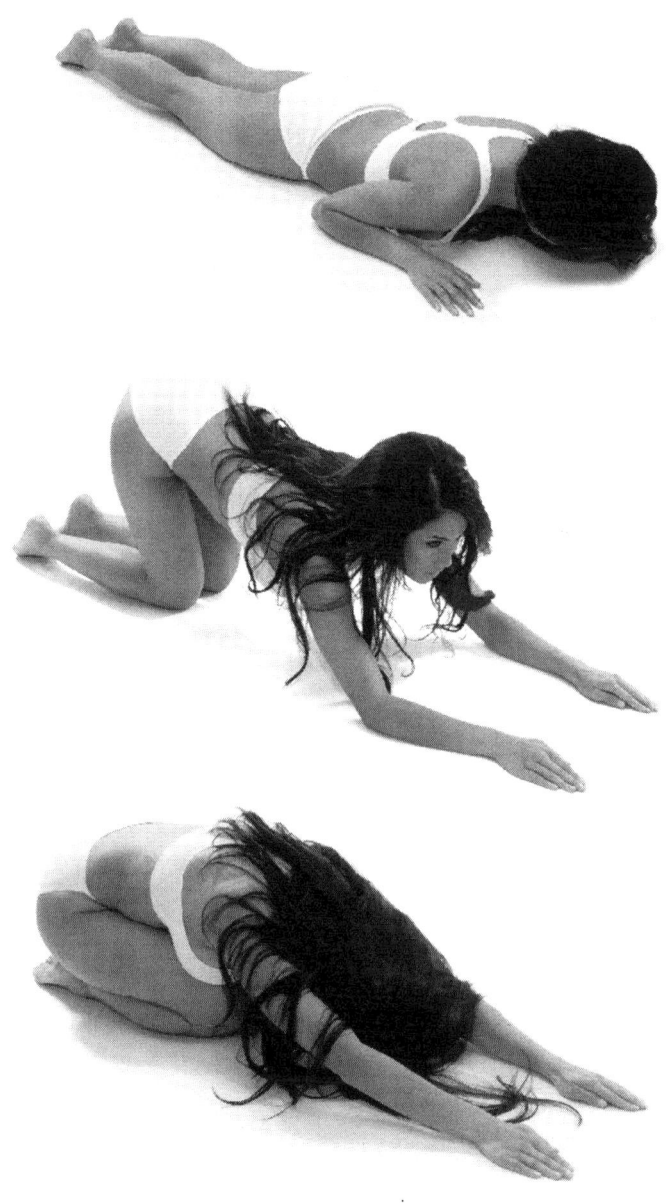

10 sec Humping
12 sec Mean Pussycat
10 sec Humping
12 sec Mean Pussycat

$= 44 \text{ sec!}$

HERE KITTY KITTY KITTY

There exists an ancient back move that has a useful application in alleviating low back pain. This move has many different names, depending on the discipline naming it. The most popular of all is the Yogis, who call it the "Mad Cat."

The Mad Cat is quite the Mr. Mistoffelees magical cat performance. The Mad Cat first gets on all fours and then cycles back and forth between a rounded "mad as hell" back, and its opposite "so happy to see you" pose with its kitty butt stuck out and up and its back and belly hanging down and low. When kitty suddenly senses a dog nearby, upsetting his feline aura, he then rounds his back, ready to charge forward. I have given the Mad Cat a bit of anger management and turned it into a more cowed "Mean Pussycat."

The Mean Pussycat is a slightly modified Mad Cat position. Starting from the "kneeling-on-all-fours" position, you lean way back and hold the pose for a count of twelve seconds, one for each letter (m-e-a-n-p-u-s-s-y-c-a-t). If you've ever slept with a dog before, then maybe you've stuck around long enough to see one stretch first thing in the morning? And canines, too, like to stretch with their front paws outstretched forward as they yawn and lean back at the same time. The Mean Pussycat takes you in the opposite direction of the sexercise moves. Think of the Mean Pussycat as your playful stretch break between your two multiples (sets) of ten humps (reps). All sexercises finish with the Mean Pussycat!

THE HABITUAL SPECTACLE WITHIN YOU

When performing your lumbar spine sexercises, you are "masterlumbating." The tempo of your humping strokes is slow-mo legato. The number of pumps per multiple is always ten. That's one per letter in the title of each sexercise. Performing the sexercise with only one multiple hump of ten is satisfactory but putting an effort into a second multiple of ten humps will give you an "A+++"—that's a perfect "A" as in perfect Ass, Agility and Abs. Two sets of ten reps with a twelve second Mean Pussycat in between is the right formula to come by. Adding this all up, if your calculations are right, your total should be forty-four seconds. What a workout, huh?

With only a forty-four second In Vitro commitment you should enjoy masterlumbating as often as you feel tension down there. It's your stretch break, your ergonomic de-stresser, and your warm beach-sand-between-toes feeling. Unloading the heavy load from the truck made you feel tense and sore? Carrying that heavy package gave you discomfort down below? Sat on your tush at work all day and having trouble getting off the chair? Tired of your morning spinal stiffy? Roll over and masterlumbate your pain away. Feeling a bit of elevator waiting rage, cell phone rage, delayed air flight rage? Lie down, relax, and watch the surprised looks you get as you masterlumbate right there on the floor. It's your spinal stress reliever, your beautiful curve provider, your disc pressure reducer, and your flexibility restorer. Do it when you feel like it, do it when you can, do it to recharge your battery, and do it before you roll over and do it again.

Masterlumbation—love it for what it is—do it for what it's worth!

DRIVING MISS CREAKY

We should have a serious discussion about car seats. They suck! All of them. Regardless of the price of the car. How many times have I heard in practice: "Oh, I have a great car seat; it's got a good low back support with a thing in it that pops out if I want it to?" How many more times have I heard: "I don't know if I can sit in my car that long" or "I can only sit for short trips now" or "I was doing fine until I had to sit in my car for three hours?" Those car facts speak louder than real Corinthian leather bucket seats.

I welcome the chance to share my car seat solutions with any mega-motor manufacturer; until then, I will continue to diagnose those "autogenic" factors in creating the worst cases of Stiffy, Sparky, Puffy and Spazzy. And by the time Creaky comes upon your back, your car will also have turned to Bedrock stone. Like owner—like car! Does your medical chart have "Toyota Syndrome," "Nissan Syndrome," or "Mercedes Syndrome" on your list of orthopedic sufferings yet? Who will invest boardroom time to help solve their sore-seated car snags?

ONE POTATO, TWO POTATO, THREE POTATO SCORE

There are four naughty sexercises, each one different from the other, based upon body positions at the start, with or without a date! Tired of reading and still not knowing what exactly you are doing when pumping, humping, pussycatting and masterlumbating? We're down to the wire. Just a bit more to learn before show and tell!

Learning the sexercise steps for one move applies to them all. They all start from a facedown position, comforted by a bed, mat, floor, or carpet underneath you. And with every peaceful and passive back rise, you will look up before you rise up. As you rise up, you will do it with your elbows bent, helping hands resting at your side at shoulder level. With every chest rise (or buttock rise), you will breath in on your way up, holding your breath at the top of your rise. At the top of your rise, the silent breath hold is held as long as it takes to say, "Hump one, hump two, hump three," after which you will release and fall back down, which finishes your first hump cycle. With every repeating rise, while rising, you will softly count to ten, not with numbers but with letters, one for each letter in the title used to describe the sexercise. And with every rise, you will demonstrate the power of control. The power of a slow-mo legato rhythm that moves softly, gently, tenderly, and ever so carefully up and down. And at the end of the pulsing torso undulations, there will be the praise of the Mean Pussycat. These are the sexercises' common denominators. Aside from these commonalities, each sexercise is unique.

11

THE SEXERCISES

It's time to make sense of all this multi-pumpy-humpy talk and put ol' humpy back together again. It's time to get humpy back into your life again. This first sexercise has the air of an ancient movement that has survived many centuries of challenge. If it is stronger than time itself, then it is stronger than you and me! It is stronger than any medical orthopedic creation. It is not "new and improved" or "modern and trendy"! Rather, it is "old and lasting," "ancient, yet good as new"!

IN VITRO SEXERCISE: XPOSED & XPLAINED: PUSH-UP AND PUMP

The two X-posed (public) and X-rated (private) sexercises are based upon this ancient movement. Perhaps you're

IN VITRO SEXERCISE: **X**POSED & PLAINED 1

THE PUSH-UP AND PUMP

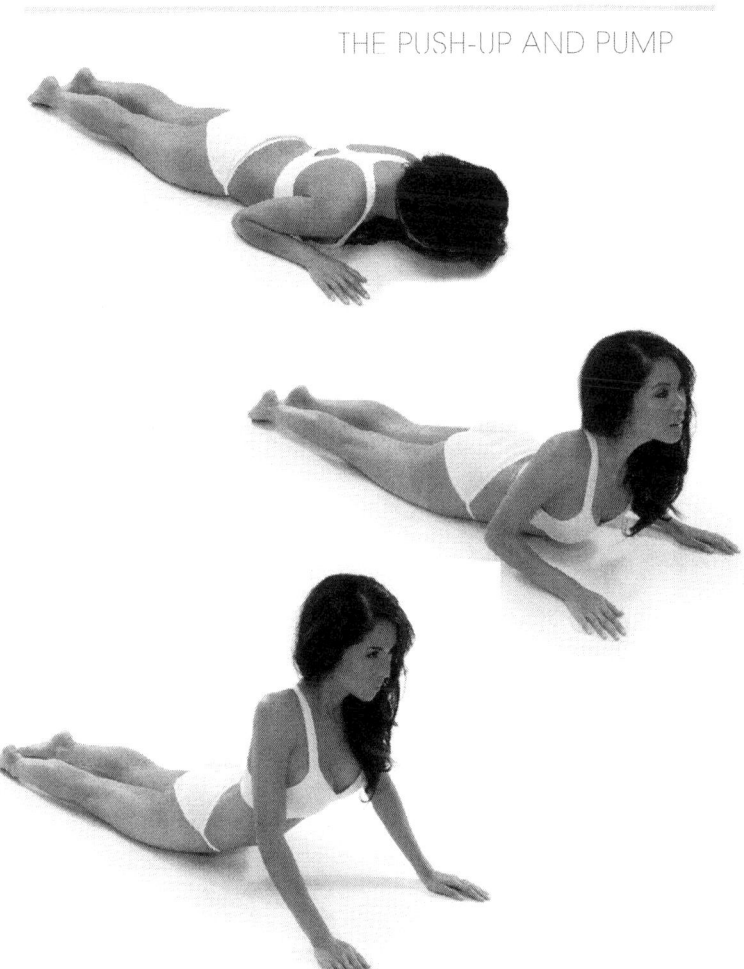

The Push-Up and Pump is this easy. Pumping up and down ten times, using each letter for every pump action.

The steady up and down motion will keep your torso in rhythm, reaching your personal maximal Torso Curve at the top of the push-up. With your breath held on the way up, your Torso Hoop is activated, keeping you safe, strong, and sexy. Remember that you should do two multiples of Push-Up and Pump, followed by the Mean Pussycat stretch. So that's Push-Up and Pump, the Mean Pussycat, followed by another multiple of Push-Up and Pump, with a final closing stretch with the Mean Pussycat. Those Torso Curves are coming back already! They've never looked better!

IN VITRO SEXERCISE: XPOSED & XPLAINED: NOSE DIVING

The second part of In Vitro's exposed is a sexercise designed to re-build hoop dreams, a sexy washboard stomach and rippling low back muscles. Although this sexercise touches upon all parts of The Terrific Torso Threesome, it pays particular attention to Torso Hoop. Hoop is the challenge in this sexercise.

Think of this move as the training program for your spinal strength, spinal stamina, and spinal erection! It's all in the hoop, baby!

It takes contractual energy (muscle work, not lawyer work!) to lift your buttock off the ground when lying face down. Although the beautiful low back curve creations are the same as the Push-Up and Pump sexercise, your lifting energy comes from your erectors, the muscles that create and maintain your torso's erection. It's the same when lifting your legs off the ground when lying face down, using

IN VITRO SEXERCISE: **X**POSED & PLAINED 2

NOSE DIVE

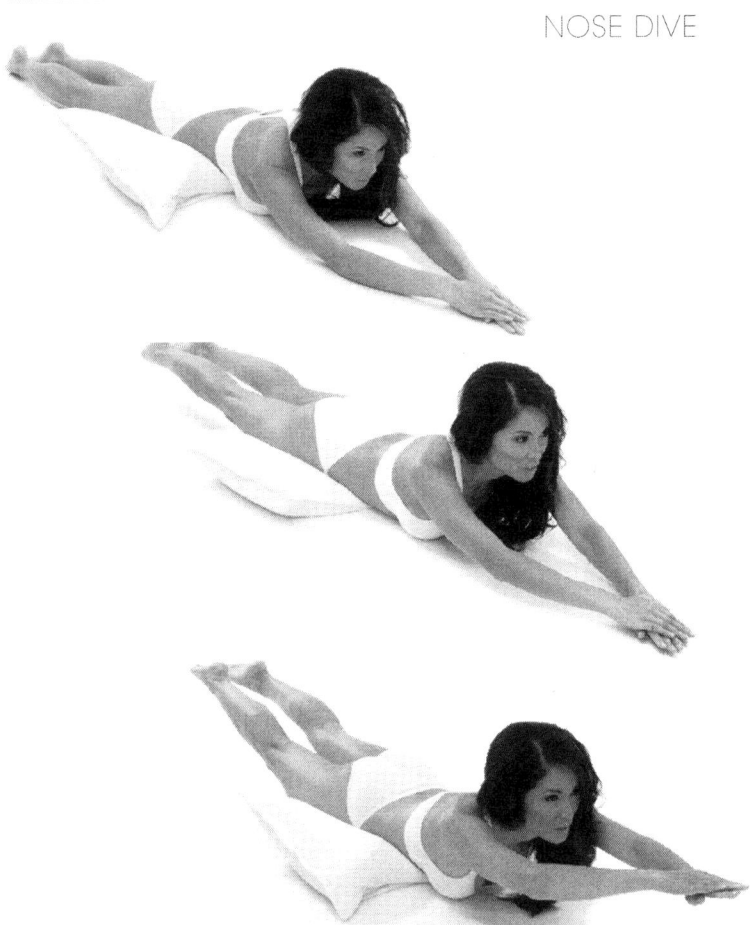

This up and down slow-mo legato motion not only keeps your torso in rhythm and torso curves looking nice, it trains your torso hoopers too.

familiar with the "Passive Push-Up." That's just the beginning of the name-calling. Yogis call it the "Cobra," super Yogis call it "Bujanga," lacto-ovo veggies call it the "Canoe," lazy asses call it the "Lazy Push-Up," aerobics enthusiasts call it the "Modified Push-Up," muscle-heads call it the "Girly Push-Up" (real men don't do half push-ups—at least not in the gym), insomniacs call it the "Morning Sunrise" and early risers call it the "Morning Salutation." I humbly call my sexercise the "Push-Up and Pump." It's the first of the next four sexercises you are about to learn and it's the one that the other three are based on.

Jack, lie face down, it's time to get pushy. With your head looking up, hands at shoulder level, hold your breath and push yourself up, up, up until you feel a tightness in your low back. Push yourself up until there is no more give, to the point right before your belt comes off the floor. Hold your breath, Jack, counting hump one, hump two, hump three, and down you go again. Good work, Jack! You go, bud! You just got over your very first hump! Don't forget to say "P" on your way down. Now pump it up again one more time. Hold it up, counting hump one, hump two, hump three, and down you go again. This time, say "U" on your way down. Pump it up one more time, Jack, calling this one "S" on the way down. Repeat these Push-Up and Pump cycles until you've completely spelled all ten letters in Push-Up and Pump. After finishing your ten Push-Up and Pump sexercise humps, take it back, relax, and get into the Mean Pussycat.

The Push-Up and Pump is this easy. Pumping up and down ten times, using each letter for every pump action.

additional helpers like your buttock muscles to lift your legs up. When pushing up and pumping (sexercise Xposed-1), the contractual energy source comes from your pecs and triceps. When you're left armless in a leg or buttock liftoff, you need low back muscle energy and abdominal isometrics. The abdominals are contracting so that your gut gets to lift off the floor too. This sexercise is also a low back strength and tone builder. With your arms still at the side to help you with your up and down moves, raise your legs while keeping your knees straight. I call this sexercise "Nose Diving." Although not described in this part of the program, you can actually go all the way and perform this sexercise with arms in front of you, ready to break water as you nose dive.

Get down, Jill, get down, and then flex. With your head looking up, hands down at your sides, hold your breath, tighten your sexy belly and push-up while at the same time, lifting your entire legs off the floor, keeping your knees straight. push-up, up, up, until you feel a tightness and hardness in your low back and tush. push-up until there is no more give, to the point right before your belt comes off the ground. Still holding your breath, count hump one, hump two, hump three, and down you go. Hope you remembered to say "N" on your way down. Now pump it up one more time, calling your second rise and fall "O." Repeat until you've spelled "Nose Diving" in its entirety, and then finish with the Mean Pussycat. The up and down slow-mo legato motion not only keeps your torso in rhythm and torso curves looking nice, it trains your torso hoopers too. Remember that you should do two multiples of ten

Nose Diving humps with the Mean Pussycat stretch after each multiple.

Don't push yourself with this second "Nose Diving" part of the Xposed-2 sexercise. It's okay if it takes a long time to get to this sexercise level. And when you decide to take on the Nose Diving sexercise, not forgetting about the Mean Pussycat breaks, only do one multiple of ten humps the first time. It's a safe way to determine if this much Nose Diving is too much in one lie-down. Muscles and bones are not re-built in one easy lie-down.

Whoever said that you couldn't have fun when in the company of yourself? Add a bit of promise to all this floor play ("If you do it, I will teach you how to get more sex into your life"—"If you do this, it'll make you as erogenous as Eros!") and just maybe you will start spending time sexercising rather than on-line Internet cruising. These next two sexercises are closer to the real thing in that they prepare you for In Vivo action. They are classified as X-rated sexercises because Torso Curve and Torso Rhythm are both bottom driven. Unless you want to give the impression you're the type who left his trench coat in the locker room, it is suggested that X-Rated sexercises be performed during "home alone" time.

IN VITRO SEXERCISES: X-RATED & PRIVATE:
CLIMB AND GRIND

As with the Xposed-1 and 2 sexercises, the first X-Rated-1 is very passive in comparison to X-Rated-2. The passivity of In Vitro's X-Rated-1 sexercise involves the working of

IN VITRO SEXERCISE: X RATED & PRIVATE 1

CLIMB & GRIND

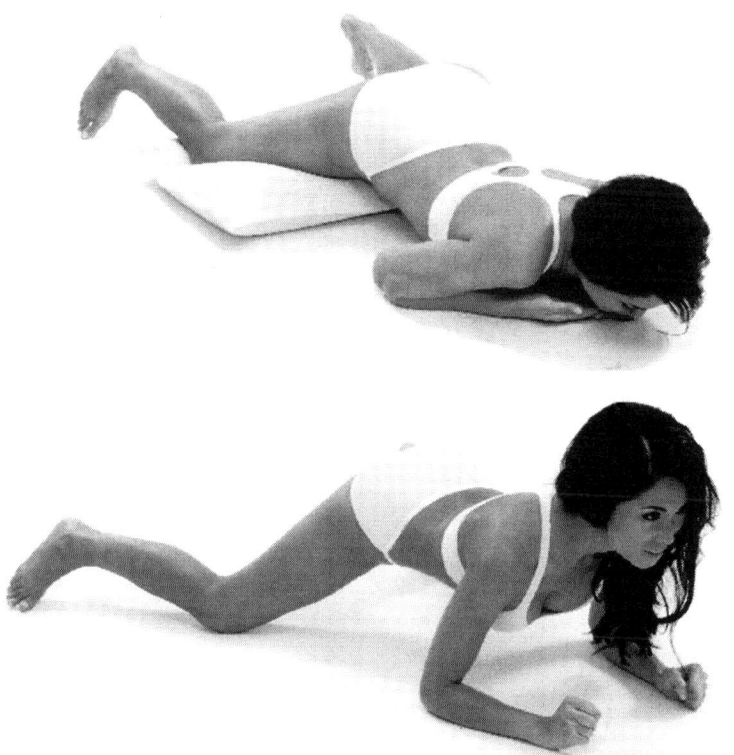

With all this climbing and grinding, if you hear the tiniest sounds of a headboard banging, you are doing something very wrong. The more headboard banging, the more your giddy-ups are simply relying too heavily on your upper body

Torso Curve and Rhythm, with minor Torso Hoop participation. It is perfectly acceptable, as with the Xposed-1 and 2 series, to never get to second base (X-Rated-2). You can still expect positive back results with minimal X-Rated-1 participation.

See Jack hump? Hump, Jack, hump! Lie face down on a pillow, legs spread, knees bent a bit, toes pointing outward. From above, your legs should look like a frog about to kick. With your eyes only looking up ahead, breathing at your normal excited rate, with the soothing and controlled legato tempo, flatten your back, tucking in as though trying to bring your knees to your chest. In other words, grind your groin into the pillow under your torso. At the same time tuck your butt in like you are doing a facedown pelvic tilt. One last push down using your entire lower torso, from belly button to pubic bone (the part that touches your bicycle's crossbar when standing), you tuck your pelvis in as tightly as you can. Crush, plush fluff, crush! And now, release your maxi-flexed pelvis, letting go of your forward thrust. While releasing your flexed pelvis, hold your breath, look up, and arch back, buttock high in the air, tailbone to the heavens, holding it at its top, counting hump one, hump two, hump three, and then releasing to complete this first hump cycle. Don't forget to say "C" on your buttock's way down for hump two. That's "C" for "Climb and Grind," the name I have given to the X-rated R-1 sexercise of the In Vitro program. It feels like you're climbing and grinding, doesn't it? This is an excellent solo exercise that requires ultimate concentration and controlled body moves. With one pelvic cycle per hump, you have ten humps to perform, one for each letter. So that's two Climb and Grind multiples with a stretching Mean Pussycat after each Climb and Grind multiple.

POLITICALLY CORRECT HUMP

With all this climbing and grinding, if you hear the tiniest sounds of a headboard banging, you are doing something very wrong. The more headboard banging, the more your giddy-ups are simply relying too heavily on your upper body. High performers don't headboard bang! With proper pelvic movement (lots of pelvic rhythm and lots of torso curvatures), you get minimal drywall damage, not to mention a safeguard against primary concussions.

IN VITRO SEXERCISE: X-RATED & PRIVATE: SPREAD & GO UP

The last sexercise is not the most important but it is, however, the sexiest of all. And it is, at the same time, the most grueling, growling, and gawking provoker. Dare to do it for stares! Although it is best performed in private session segments, I personally don't have a problem performing X-Rated-2 for the dilated pupils of gawking public eyes. All eyes on me! "Just what is he doing down there?" Well, if you don't know, then you're not one of us, are you?

Take over, Jill. Lay that adrenaline pumped frame of yours down there, face down; as you lie there, arms at your side, you look up, pulmonary rhythmics and thumping cardiacs massaging the ground below you, your beautiful

X RATED & PRIVATE 2

SPREAD & GO UP

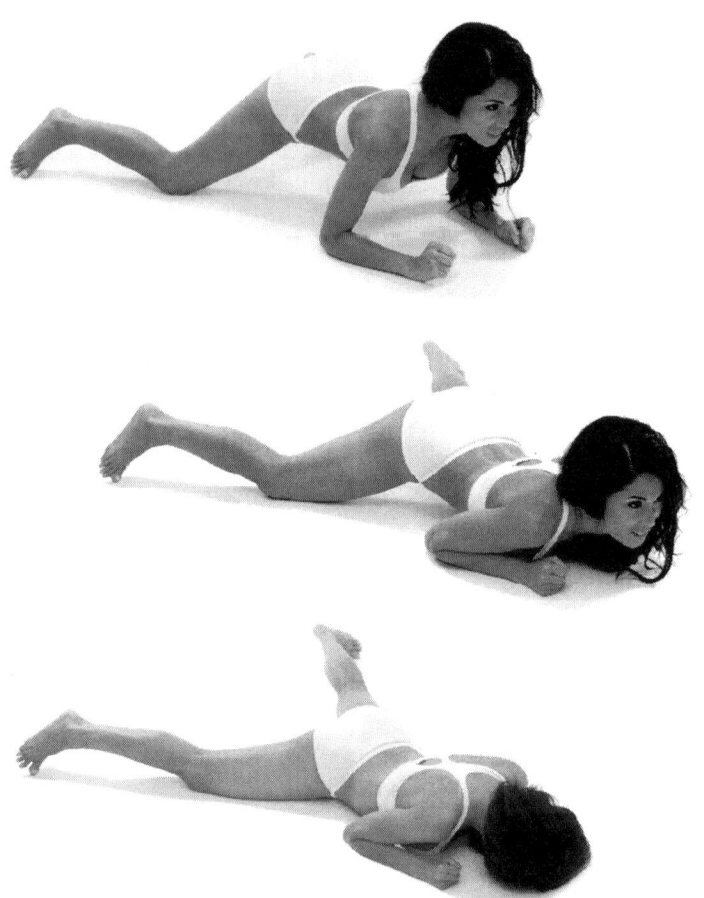

All eyes on me! "Just what is he doing down there?
"Well, if you don't know, then you're not one of us, are you?

long legs spread apart, knees bent like a horny toad ready to whip kick your way to the other side of the singles pond where he-toads croak. Hold your breath, Jill, tighten your sexy belly and push yourself up off the ground while keeping your knees bent. Only she-knees and she-elbows should be touching the surface underneath you, Jill. Legs are in the same position as the Climb & Grind sexercise. Hold up, hump one, hump two, hump three! Good work, Jill!

Now drop yourself all the way down with a commanding "Climb and Grind"—type of pelvic thrust, one last back flattening thrust, belly bones to pubic buttons and all. How the ground loves your pulses, Jill, massaged by your rhythmic breaths and cardiac metrics. The ground-squishing belly bone movement completes a cycle. Cry-out "S," Jill…not for sexy, not for screams of passion, not for sizzling action, not for steamy hot, and not for "Seventh Heaven" either! Cry-out "S" for "Spread and Go Up." This is the name I have given to the X-Rated-2 sexercise.

Work your way up to being able to perform two multiples of ten Spread and Go-Up humps, one hump for each letter. Remember to finish each Spread and Go-Up multiple with a well-deserved Mean Pussycat stretch. Your mission is to Spread and Go-Up twice, with the Mean Pussycat stretch in between each multiple.

THE IN VITRO SYNOPSIS

Push-Up and Pump: Xposed-1—Adult Accompaniment: Exposed

- Two multiples of Push-Up and Pump, with the Mean Pussycat after each multiple;

Nose Diving: Xposed-2—Adult Accompaniment: Exposed
- Two multiples of Nose Diving, with the Mean Pussycat after each multiple;

Climb and Grind: X-Rated-1—Private
- Two multiples of Climb and Grind, with the Mean Pussycat after each multiple;

Spread and Go Up: X-Rated-2—Private
- Two multiples of Spread and Go Up, with the Mean Pussycat after each multiple.

12

GETTING' KISSY KISSY WITH SEXING

There remains a bit more to discover before you're ready to share your newfound treasure. Having become a connoisseur of sexercises, it is time to give you the savoir faire of In Vivo action.

In Vitro was designed for when it is just about you, in the lab, while In Vivo is real life! In Vivo is vivifying action that can only happen when there are two. Viva la Vivo! In Vivo is duo action that heals by using the powers generated from the sharing of two sexual souls...the third very powerful healing source of the program (see Doctrinaire Disclaimers).

A-B-CHI

Sex Chi is the soul of one's sexual energy. We all have a Sex Chi. Touched by the right one, in the right way, someone's Sex Chi will make you feel good. You feel it…something. One Sex Chi soul gives off Sex Chi energy to the other soul. Good Sex Chi feeds your feel. Sex Chi is alive and can be transferred with passionate physical touching, with the gentleness of communicating minds, and with the use of sensual senses. Good Sex Chi has the power to shake the senses right out of you. Chi is what your sex is all about. How much Chi are you sharing when you're involved?

Loner or party-goer, partnered or single, "seducee" or seducer, hunter or hunted, all man or whole woman, suffering patient or healer sexician, what goes on remains the same. The energies! The moment! The gravity! The Chi! The heat! Marvin Gay's "Sexual Healing" playing in your head— "Let's make love tonight, 'cause you do it right! When I get this feeling, I need sexual healing!" Anyone who chooses to go the In Vivo way fits into the equation somewhere. Souls will meet and energies will be exchanged through sex. Chis connect. Sex for love, sex for sport, sex for healing, sex!

While going through the motions of learning about "healing through intimate touch," you must always involve The Torso Threesome. If you want therapy through pleasure and pleasure through therapy, Torso Curve, Rhythm, and Hoop can never be forgotten when passionately involved. Sex that heals must rely heavily on The Torso Threesome. You cannot turn your back on the existence of the symbiosis between the three torso models—not if therapy and liberty are expected benefits. Encouraging those curves to arch themselves into a blissful position of lowered disc pressure, continuously moving those curves in a slow-mo legato rhythm, and training those hoopers to contract hard to protect the vulnerable torso interiors are the three applications you must learn if you want to fix a necrophiliac spine. Knowing about and knowing the feel of The Torso Threesome is a must. Satisfaction will be guaranteed, not only from knowing the location of all the pleasure parts, but also from knowing the feel of a curveless torso, a motionless torso, and an unprotected and weakened torso. Go ahead, feel your own, test your own, look around you, touch a friend's, help a partner!

SO MANY ZENS, SO LITTLE TIME

Eeny Meany Spiny Mo! So Many Spines, So Little Time! So many positions to pick from and so many bad ones to pick on, too! Tangles and knots, figures and fissures, dominances and passivities, pleasure givings and pleasure receivings, touches and feels, stretchers and strengtheners—should there be only one way? Favorite positions do exist, but you've got to know the rules first. Once you know the rules of the Sexy Back game, you can go out there in the playing fields of singlehood to see how good you are at playing the sex therapy game. Rules are more than enforceable instructions; they are the tenets of good back (and good sex) health. The Rules add up to the Sextitution!

The Sextitution is what you first learn before mounting the In Vivo program. It proclaims the rights of a sufferer, the consents of the givers, the governing powers of the spine, the limits of the seductions, the laws governing the actions, the civility of nervous advancements, and the realization of a dream. The Sextitution is a code of ethics: a prayer, a mission statement, and a purpose that helps keep your world back-pain-free and full of sexual opportunities. If you understand and live by the Sextitution, then you are ready to get it on. If you obey the law enforcement guidelines, then only good things will come your way!

THE SEXTITUTION

We, the people, in order to form a more perfect and therapeutic union, will establish amongst ourselves, In Vivo with our partners, the Sextitution articles for the purpose of:

a) "spinal justice" for both our bad backs, and for our whole selves;

b) "tranquility" for both our bad backs and for our whole selves; and

c) "common defense" for both our bad backs and for our whole selves.

We, the people, will assist with the promotion of general welfare, and secure the blessing of liberty to our spinal selves and whole being. We, the people, will ordain, establish, and live by the articles of the Sextitution for sex and for our long living Spine. In Vivo we trust!

THE 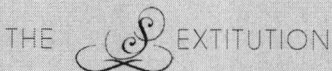EXTITUTION

Article One of the Sextitution 1.0

We, the People, will live by the grounded premise that Torso Curve, Rhythm, and Hoop must be met for safety and therapeutic benefit, for ourselves, and for the people we love. Sexercise is Medicine!

Article Two of the Sextitution 2.0

We, the people, will live by the respectful virtues of:

- 2.01 Patience, to allow for natural healing. Our justice delayed was justice denied; patience is therefore the penitence for delays (the delay in taking care of our backs);
- 2.02 Focus, the virtue that will provide maximum results with a minimal program approach. We understand that In Vitro and In Vivo are the affectionately abbreviated versions of what could have been lengthy and complex;
- 2.03 Hardiness, as nothing worthy is ever free, and escaping the sufferings in our recovery, the pains for our gains, is simply not viable. We understand and respect "reality healing."

Article Three of the Sextitution 3.0

We, the people, understand that In Vitro and In Vivo programs are not exercises as much as back savior sexercises and sexing attitudes. They are back care moves, and like the grooming duties of our beings, we will add In Vitro and In Vivo to our everyday grooming tasks.

Article Four of the Sextitution 4.0

We, the people, live in a society where bones rule. We will respect The Torso Threesome bone rules because bones rule! We will seek to maximize motor neuron excitability (increased muscle power as a result of increased nerve voltage power to the muscle) with In Vitro sexercises and In Vivo sexing. We must respect the dangers that our modernized society has inflicted upon our spinal agility, asses, and abdominals.

Article Five of the Sextitution 5.0

We, the people, will obtain an informed consent before establishing any physical contact, as healer or partner. If permission to come aboard is not given, then we will turn ourselves over to the healing powers of In Vitro therapeutics.

Article Six of the Sextitution 6.0

We, the people, in the practical application of In Vivo, accept that justice equates only with sexual orgasmic endings. Justice prevails only when both In

Vivo parties have climbed, reached, and planted their personal Coat of Arms on the summit of their organic internal combustion. Satisfaction must be a surefire guarantee.

Article Seven of the Sextitution 7.0

We, the people, have, men and women alike, souls of equal weight. Both genders, therefore, must give way to the suffering one. It is the suffering soul who will hold sway over the superior seat, selecting top as the most therapeutic position. In Vivo, we believe that XY=XX!

Article Eight of the Sextitution 8.0

In the event of rushed pleasures, we, the people, will still begin with one ceremonious warm-up multiple of the Push-Up and Go-Up kind, followed by only one Mean Pussycat. This ceremonial movement can be done alone or with our In Vivo partner beneath us.

Article Nine of the Sextitution 9.0

We, the people, will learn the In Vitro sexercises and shall apply the In Vitro methods to In Vivo therapy while honoring the following subsections:
- 9.01 In Vitro's X-rated sexercises closely simulate "the real thing." In Vivo, we will perform

legato multiples of Climb and Grind movements, with, if manageable, the occasional
controlled diving move into a very relaxed
Mean Pussycat;

- 9.02 For strengthening therapeutics, we will
  progress to the ultimate action move, the
  Spread and Go-Up move, with all its back
  muscle power and torso hooping abdominal
  contractions. Not more than three multiples
  of ten humps are to be performed in one lie-
  down, with the stretching Mean Pussycat move
  in between multiples; this level of contracting
  intensity is to be alternated with multiples of
  the more passive Climb and Grind sexercise
  move, keeping in mind to occasionally dive
  down into the Mean Pussycat pose;

- 9.03 When adventuring into the wilderness
  of "acrobatomania," leaving behind missionary
  limits, we, the people, will keep in mind
  The Torso Threesome sex-guide. We will favor
  a beautiful and sexy Torso Curve, we will
  keep with a controlled Torso Rhythm,
  and we will hold the isometric abdominal
  wall contractions to maximize Torso Hoop,
  regardless of the "sexacrobatomaniacal"
  positions we take. We, the people, will be

guided by The Torso Threesome and we will carefully apply the threesome to all positions encouraged by the heat of our moments, making the necessary alterations if the Torso Threesome components cannot be met.

Article Ten of the Sextitution 10.0

We, the people, will form a perfect union, embracing our physical, mental, and spiritual individualities.

MACK THE BACK MAN

It's a new night! This time, Jill isn't going to pick a locked-up Jack to help fix her spinal ails. Living under spinal duress is not going to be her life. Jill was very tired of her last desperate measures. It had become so irksome to answer all the calls she'd received from her ad that read: "Wanted: meaningless overnight relationship to help heal a suffering girl's single spine." Imagine the hefty sum of incoming calls she had to return. No Siree, she thought. This time, I'm going to do it right.

Relying heavily on The Sisy Squat Sex Test, if her pick even came close to losing his balance on his way down, the victim wasn't even going to get an invitation off the floor, let alone back to her nest. The "how to" in approaching her man became so much easier when she started using her Sisy Squat challenge as the ice-breaker. Thanks to The Sisy Squat trick at hand, turning talented tricks was now effortless for the sexy siren. Until the advent of the Sexy Back, she never knew if she would be sleeping with the enemy... until she actually was!

Not two seconds after her grand entrance into the bar, she saw him. The Mack she picked out was built thick, looked strong as a buck and as eager as a beaver, ready for his turn at some hump luck. She could tell by looking through the tight-knit sweater he was sporting that this Mack's waistline was certainly holding no water. No gut. Nice butt. And those low back lumps of his—those weren't back fat, either. Jill knew that underneath this knit was a "bod" with low back muscles so ripped that the skin looked like a Christmas tree. You could see in Jill's face the look of a proud hunter's find. You could almost hear her inner dialogue through Springsteen's jamming coming from the jukebox: Ripped bulging backs and rippled flat abs...just what the doctor ordered!

When he leaned over the bar for a fair grab of bar nuts, you could see his back steaks making two parallel bumps on the back of his shirt. It was like he was keeping two boat fenders back there; two mounds with a crevice in between them deep enough to hide a 10BC fire extinguisher. Unknowingly, the Mack passed The Sisy Squat Sex Test with flying colors and got his invitation back to Jill's flat faster than it took him to get back up to her eye level. Poor Jill, her luck had not been good lately, which is why her Chi was so desperate for some feeding. Nothing a good night with Mack couldn't fix.

It was her back, her place, her invitation, and tonight, she was determined to stay in control. Jill knew the rules and Mack didn't know there were any! Although she preferred to keep the details of her intentions to herself, the Mack didn't look like he would probably care if he ever found out he was being bamboozled into an evening of therapeutic sex.

"On your back, Big Mack!" she commanded as she pushed him down and laid herself flat on top of her muscle man, with her hands on the bed next to his baboon shoulders. He tried to make lingual connections but she turned away, her eyes looking up and to the right, like she was thinking about something mathematically important. Looking up too, Jack caught sight of the notches on the ol' proverbial bedpost. He knew perfectly well that those weren't decorative Louis XIV bedpost carvings. She let him grab hold of her tush, and like a howling wolverine, she raised herself up, head still cocked back, with only a short grunt coming from her throat as she held her breath and tightened her torso. Up and down she went, as Mack lay there, enjoying the tactile groping of her soft gluteal epidermis and the rhythmical peeps, peeks, and pops of her excited mammary mounds. The grunts she made as she held her breath on her way up, tightening her perfecto torso she-curves, were tightly connected to Mack's auditory nerve to parasympathetic pubic stimulators (medical talk for...boing!!! A transverse process has risen!!!) Little Mack shifted from already gifted to an even more talented Big Mack...Jill's gift.

After ten Push-Up and Go Up humping cycles, she was feeling better already. Done with her warm-up, she got on all fours and leaned herself way back into the Mean Pussycat pose. Holy hair job! How much more could Big Mack take? Face-to-groin level, her long "Coyote Ugly" tresses floating on his washboard abs, she noticed that he was losing it from the look of his bouncing stomach ripples. Up and down they shook, like he was being tickled to his "petite mort." All she felt was the stretching release in her low back—all he could feel was a step closer to his own Mack attack. Hold yourself together, Mack, there's so much more to come!

Enough with the foreplay; Jill moves into In Vivo. Always face down, on top and in control, she needed only the passive movements of In Vivo to feed her back's hunger. This time around, she wasn't going to get into the strength-building moves. Forget the Spread and Go Up tonight! I'm all Climb and Grind with my one and only Mean Pussycat, she thought. Already feeling the change from a self-serving (Mack would disagree with "self-serving") round of ten Push-Up and Go Up's with one Mean Pussycat move, Jill was ready for Big Mack's attack. She felt that she was in good hands this time—ten comforting Mack digits roaming all over her tension-free tail, and ten digits of her own scanning every inch of the beast. Since one Push-Up and Go Up warm-up was enough for Jill, it was time for booty action. Mack's Big Mack looked like it had been shocked with Viagra paddles.

Ready, willing, and waiting for Jill's dominant touch, Mack wanted in bad, and she was so close to letting it all happen. Steadfastly fixing her upper torso onto Mack's, she began to crush his lower torso, deeply swallowing it into her warm and comfy interior. Mack caught on fast, pulling Jill's glutes closer to him. His grip was strong, her forward thrust was inviting. Mack, well, is just happy right now; Jill, well, is just glad it's not Jack below her this time around. With legato slow-mo style, like moving in warm honey, Jill's bottom pulled away from Mack. Arching back, buttock lifting off the Mack, her Torso Curve appeared—a beautiful back valley between two mountain peaks named after her beauties: "Upper Back" and "Buttock Peaks." The silhouette of these twin peaks brought Mack closer to his own peak. Mack could feel her breath sucking in and holding it, which tightened her belly. Mack felt her rigidity; he knew she was getting ready again for another humping cycle. Looking up above her head, eyes rolled up at that same thinking spot again; he felt as though she was ready to plunge back into him and suck away his entire energy. That's only one cycle. Can Mack last? Jill releases her breath, looks into Mack's eyes as she pulls herself closer to him. How much longer could Mack hold off? He heard a whispered sound from Jill, sounds of a soft spell brushing the skin of his wet neck. He felt her chin movements on his jugular. The magic spell stimulated his eardrum, hearing her whispering only one word: "Sea." Sea? Mack had no idea just how much of his Sex Chi he was giving Jill, the honeybee queen of all Succubi.

BIG MACK'S SECOND ATTACK

Jill's back had been freaking out on her more and more lately. Too much back-busting hill climbing, she guessed. She knew that she had to do more for her back so that she could last longer in between the sexercise sessions with her now-steady boyfriend, Mack. The Climb and Grind moves were good, but she had to give in to the Spread and Go Up moves if she wanted to get stronger. Now was the time because Mack's Sex Chi was right for her.

On Mack's next visit Jill was ready to do more than the usual passive masterlumbation grind with her new steady "friend." Three multiples of ten humps of Spread and Go Up were what she was going to do. She was going to have herself a sex sweat this time around.

Her routine started with the same warm-up events, one multiple of Push-Up and Go Up followed by the Mean

Pussycat. Mack loved Jill's "Coyote hair jobs," tickling his nether region as she held her Mean Pussycat pose. But this time, their get-together was going to be different. The usual Push-Up and Go Up passive sex play was going to be preceded by hot active sex play.

Still on top of Mack, her thigh squeeze was much tighter and higher, squeezing Mack's torso with her knees. Straddling Mack, she ground her pelvis down onto what she had now nicknamed "Jilly's Big Mack."

This was a tougher move for Jill, but with the help of a little grunt and a lot of abdominal hooper strength, it was pleasing Mack to no end. She released her crushing grind on the Big Mack, and started with the out-and-out uprising movement. Howling, she pushed herself up, away from Mack's chest. Her Torso Curve was all there, as well as her "hard as rock" torso erectors and torso abdominals that looked as flat and tight as, well, Mack's own. Torso Hoop was maxed out and she was moving steady with a slow-mo Torso Rhythm.

Pushing up, grunting it out, she used those chest and triceps muscles to reach the peak of her rise. She then let it all go down, allowing all of him to get closer and deeper as she fell back on top of Mack. Her exhalation released a soft whisper that sounded to Mack like a soft "yes.". Poor Mack still didn't know what was going on with Jill and she wasn't going to let him go until her two Spread and Go Up multiples were completed. After three multiples and purry little Mean Pussycat hair jobs, Mack, too, was finished.

NOT A SCRATCH ON THEM OR YOU!

Oh yeah! How your world has changed! If you read all the instructions right, then you will have exciting new horizons ahead of you. You may never think of sex the same way again! Never again will you have to pay attention to those "better sex" video 'zine ads—you know, the ones that always catch your eye long enough to at least make you bend the page corner for future reference. "Not me, honey, the magazine must have fallen on that page!" Oh yeah? Then how come the page corner was bent when she found it?

Talk about the program with others, encourage them to get involved, and get excited about it with others, too. Open their world! Introduce yourself and tell them about the discovery of your new-found healing science using "cupism" as the icebreaker. Who knows, maybe one thing will lead to another. With the sharing of your sexual soul may come the discovery of a soulmate! The soul who mates may encounter a lifetime soulmate twosome. Don't give up hope on the possibilities of romance. The beauty of this program is not only about its back-fixing properties. Its methods provide a charming entrance into someone's life. Learn to recognize if other "spinomaniacs" like you are involved with the program. They will have nice-looking Torso Curves. They will know how to move while keeping with the rhythm and curve of their torso. Their involvement with the Sexy Back program may even be publicly exposed when practicing the sexercise moves in out-in-the-open places like the gym. Approach, greet, acknowledge, and hopefully touch down! Don't be shy! If you're a lonely solo who would rather go In Vivo, then look, and you shall find!

Four In Vitro sexercises, two In Vivo moves, one Sextitution—I think that's enough! You have all the makings of a perfect recipe to fix the chronic back pain that is very likely the result of The Guilty Triad (no agility, no ass and no abs). You've been told about The Torso Threesome (Torso Curve, Torso Rhythm, and Torso Hoop). You now have the "know-how" to know what's safe, what's risky, and what's just plain thick when it comes to putting your body in positions that will compromise the integrity of your back bones and back meat!

With only two In Vivo positions that favor four important mechanical concepts that will fix your back (the restoration of lumbar mobility, the improvement of bone position, the reduction of disc pressure, and the strengthening of low back muscles), these bare essentials were "the ones" picked for the Sexy Back program. "The one" In Vivo move is passive and has corrective effect. "The other one" is preventative and has constructive benefits. Corrective touches upon pain, and preventative touches upon re-strengthening. Think of corrective as allopathic medicine. The western medical mind likes to put things off, while the eastern medical mind is more preventative. The program wthinking blocks that will help you know what's safe, and what's "ballsy" for your back.

EXAMINING ALL OPTIONS

Let's have a little fun! It's time to put your knowledge to the test. Let's see if you've learned to recognize when you are compromising your back. Although the applications you've learned universally apply to all environments (out of bed, as much as in), we will keep with the theme and continue to challenge your skills by testing your talents in the bedroom—safety talents, that is. The back-fixing sexy bedroom moves you've learned are more dynamic than the conventional "mono-metric" action moves. Mono-metric is defined as a movement that does not change in direction or position—yawn!

The beauty of In Vivo is in its design...combining "multi-metric" movement with the smoothness and beauty of a dancing human form. In Vivo becomes an art of human movement, combining a sequence of body movements. These sexy multi-metric movements are specifically designed to help deal with the inherent back problems at hand. They have a purpose, remember? (Not to say that the mono-metric yawns don't, either!)

The typical "joyus sexis" positions are static mono-metric positions that are simply held in place until either a body part goes numb, house maid's knees act up, toe nail beds turn blue, or cell phones ring. Your Sexy Back program's knowledge will be tested with your analysis of fifteen mono-metric sexual positions. Let's see just how good your sexician diagnostic skills are.

THE FINE PRINT

Fifteen mono-metric positions will be described. We will use the world's most famous couple as models: Jack for he and Jill for she. In this examination, you will only have to pick from "safe" or "not safe." Since there are two people for each mono-metric position, a perfect score will therefore be thirty out of thirty.

Here are cheat notes that will help make things easier for you: always investigate Torso Curve (What position is the body stuck in, lordotic or alordotic? Does the body have the freedom to shift back and forth?), Torso Rhythm (When he's in this position, does he look like he's got a bad case of El Rigor Mortis? Will she move at all if you poke her? Can you cycle back and forth to keep from seizing?), and Torso Hoop (Does this position look like it could be a good abdominal workout at the same time? Are the abdominal muscles involved in this move? How much force does gravity play in this position?). For each position, investigate all three factors, paying particular attention to the first two torso concepts discussed above.

To answer the dangerous questions correctly, you simply have to say "yes—it's safe" or "no—it's a crazy move, what were they thinking?'" Give yourself a point for every right answer. Hope you have sexician's medical malpractice insurance.

You need seventy percent to pass (that's twenty one out of thirty). Why seventy? When I was in medical school (not that long ago) seventy was the passing mark. Besides, would you put yourself in the hands of a sexician who happens to have passed with a borderline fifty percent mark? If the sexual attraction is strong, then probably so! But you still need a seventy in my books to be certified! Think safety, not therapy! Good Hump Luck!

You have forty seconds to answer each question, for a total of thirty minutes to complete the test, given that you can read the entire question in ten seconds or less. Heroes, mind you, can do it in fifteen. But if you need an extra minute's grace, then take it. It's the least I can do for my adding a load of comments that had nothing to do with position descriptions. This is both a time and skill exam—killer! Good training, if you ask me. We all know that in real life, if your timing isn't right, you're not going to be going anywhere—even with all the gifted know-how in the world.

You will begin the exam by figuring out what mono-metric poses Jack and Jill are in, followed by a Jack "yes or no" and Jill "yes or no" answer. If you answer "yes," it means that the position is safe and applies no danger to his or her low back. Although the positions are mono-metric, if Jack or Jill found him or herself locked up and completely immobile, with nowhere to move, then the position will not favor Torso Rhythm. If two of the three torso principles can be applied, on a safety scale, the answer should be yes. Ready or not, the timer is on and here they come…let's get naked:

LET THE QUIZZING BEGIN!

Rodeo Cowgirl

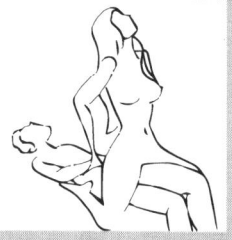

Jack is lying on his back, his lower spine slightly arched, with knees straight or bent. Jill is having most of the fun, lying on top of Jack, staring at his feet, and leaning back like she's riding a mechanical bull at a corporate Christmas party. Get the picture?

Jack   Yes / No
Jill   Yes / No

Faithful Missionaries

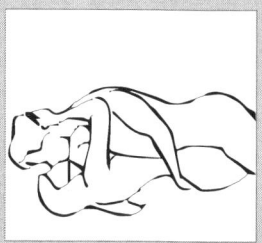

Jill is lying on her back, knees bent and legs apart to accommodate Jack, who is on top of Jill. If you can't picture this, remember to put this book back in Daddy's drawer so he won't know you were touching his things.

Jack   Yes / No
Jill   Yes / No

Side Swipin'

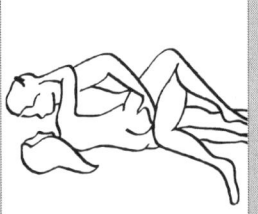

Jill is facing Jack. Both are on their sides. No leg-crushing here! Jack has his top leg between hers, and her top leg is over his. Quaint!

Jack   Yes / No
Jill   Yes / No

Crouching Mister, Hidden Dragon Lady

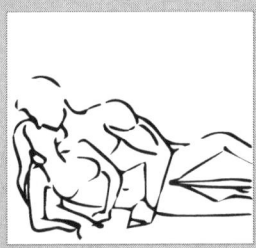

A variety to the Side Swipin' move is with Jill facing away from Jack, both lying on their sides. Crouching together with Jill's bottom leg between his and her top one over his top leg, the move is on. They both look like they're doing one serious Olympiad synchro side-stroke.

Jack   Yes / No
Jill   Yes / No

Surfboarding

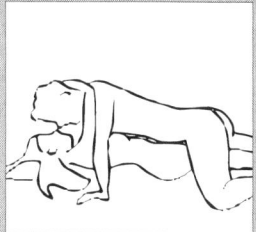

Jill is making like a surf-board—flat on her back, knees straight and legs together like she is playing Charades. "Guess what I am right now, Jack?" A surfboard, Jill, a very stiff one! And now, Jack gets to hop on top of his surfboard and make waves. He's lying on top of Jill with his legs wrapped around hers (treading water).

Jack   Yes / No

Jill   Yes / No

Fido's Pow Wow!

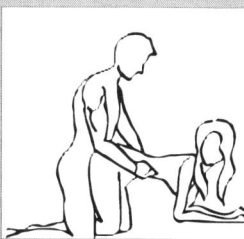

Jill is on all primal fours; Jack is all for primal fours. He's happy, kneeling right behind her. Need more be described? I think not!

Jack   Yes / No

Jill   Yes / No

The Elevate-Her Wall-Bang-Her

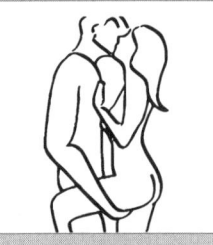

Elevator, parking garage, American Airline's powder room…if the moment is right, who cares where they are! Jack pins Jill against the wall. Leaning slightly back with legs spread a bit, knees bent, Jack's position will accommodate accurate instrumental positioning and save him from breaking his music stand in half. Jill makes like a ballerina and wraps one leg around Jack's waist.

Jack	Yes / No
Jill	Yes / No

Heimlich Man Over

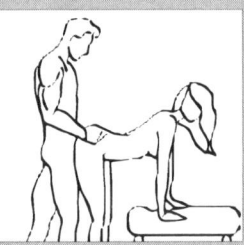

Jill looks like she's being given the Heimlich from behind, bent over an armchair, only Jack's got his hands everywhere but on her upper abdominal quadrant, where they should be if she was choking for real. Jack's legs are spread, squatting low for a perfect fit behind Jill, making sure she doesn't choke on the Big Mack.

Jack is playing macho man, with two hands on his girl at all times. Spit it out, Jill! Spit it out!

Jack   Yes / No

Jill   Yes / No

Top of the Whirl

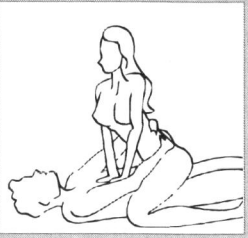

Jill is on top, facing Jack while straddling him with her knees bent and lower legs wrapped underneath his legs. She looks like she's holding him down during one of those romantic country picnic wrestles. Jack is lying flat on his back, holding onto Jill's tush. Jill braces her upper body with her arms straight and hands resting on his shoulders or chest. Jack's legs are straight, and his neck is lifted a bit to get a good view of Jill's whirlers.

Jack   Yes / No

Jill   Yes / No

The Grenade Dive

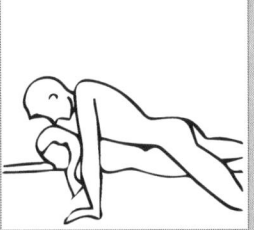

Jack is lying atop Jill like he is protecting her from a nearby grenade blast. Both are facing down. Her legs are kept together and her derrière comes up to facilitate Jack's visit. Jack is leaning on his forearms for support.

Jack   Yes / No
Jill   Yes / No

Hunk Her Down and Hunker Down

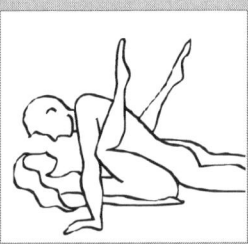

Jill is lying on her back with her knees spread and pulled very high over her chest. Jack is sitting a few inches higher than the normal Faithful Missionary joy spot. Since Jack will get tired quickly in this position, he will support himself on Jill's legs. Thanks, Jill!

Jack   Yes / No
Jill   Yes / No

Lap Whacking

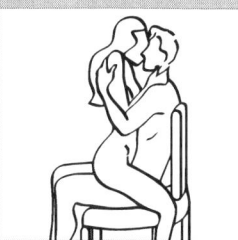

Jack is sitting in a narrow chair with his hips up a bit. Jill is straddling Jack, still on her feet, bouncing up and down like a fraternity girl at the end of her twin bed, bouncing her seat up and down on her posture-pedic. Did Jack ask you to the prom, Jill? Huh, Jill?

Jack   Yes / No
Jill   Yes / No

Jack Hammer Hams Her

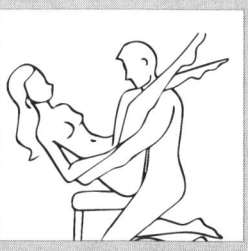

Jill is sitting on a low chair, coffee table or sofa (her favorite), leaning back with her legs wrapped around Jack's neck (well, maybe just resting on his shoulders while Jack wishes her legs were doing the neck wrapping thing). Jack is kneeling in front of Jill with his pelvis higher than Jill's. Jack occasionally gets up higher to kneel on the sofa, grabbing its back end for extra support.

Jack   Yes / No
Jill   Yes / No

Rock-A-My-Baby-On-His-Tree-Stub

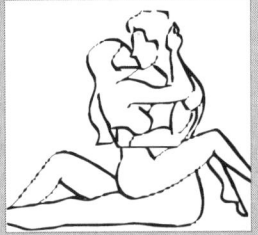

Jack is sitting at the head of the bed, his back to the board. His legs are spread, making a little potty hole for Jill to sit in. Jill's legs are wrapped around Jack, both sitting face-to-face. She is supporting herself using her hands while leaning back a bit.

     Jack   Yes / No
     Jill   Yes / No

Sling Shot Stir Ups

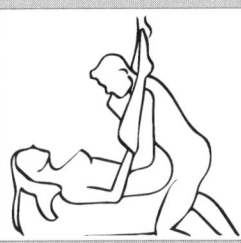

Jill is lying on a tabletop approximately one foot lower than Jack's pelvis. She's flat on her back with her pelvis tilted up, flattening her back completely on the table. Her legs are high up in the air, knees hooking onto Jack's upper arms. Jill is showing the cookie monster how to make a very big "V" using her legs. The cookie monster is leaning into Jill, crouching down for a perfect glove fit. His hands are resting all over Jill's sweet cookies.

      Jack   Yes / No

      Jill   Yes / No

Stop! Put your pencil down and record your time. Remember, should you decide to go back and change an answer, chances that your change was for the good are not on your side. For every minute over 30, you will deduct this number from your total score at the end of the examination.

ANSWERS

Rodeo Cowgirl

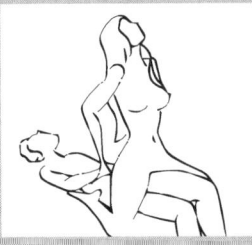

Go for it, Jack! Jill, the lucky girl, is getting her Universal Studio fix for the year. Both partners are in favorable positions. Jack's biggest problem is holding his Little Jack down in his proper position. He's also got to be careful because if Jill gets too carried away, her straddling bobbing can make his Little Jack go crack-crack. That's why Jack's job is to keep his little sailor in the right position so that he doesn't get splashed around too much. Jill, on the other hand, has good flexibility. She can cycle back and forth, leaning back and then leaning way forward for some pinky tickling. Jill will also get a good hoop workout in this position. Have fun guys! Jack, yes; Jill, Yesssssssss!

Faithful Missionary

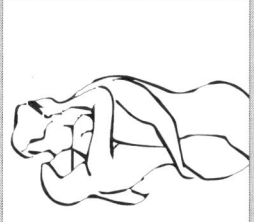

Jack will never get back pain if he sticks to this position. Jill, on the other hand, is setting herself up for some serious misery. With her pelvis flexed like that, not to mention the added weight of a few heavy potato bags on top of her, she's got nowhere to go. Jill is the villain in this "Missionary Impossible" sequel. No matter how hunky he is, a spud's a spud. She's trapped and ol' tater head is not doing much to help her out. No Torso Rhythm and her Torso Curves are completely crushed. Jack is a yes! You're the man, Jack! Jill is a no! Get out while you can, woman!

Of course, if Jack were a trained sexician, he would know to place a hand in the small of her back and move her like she's never been moved before, lifting her up and down with a passionate, yet firm grip. Jill would then be in safe hands. And if Jack really wanted to be a Harlequin dream, then he would place himself a little higher than the usual humpy spot. This way, for every Jack move, Jill's presto button gets rubbed the right way—the whole way! Jack gets a good hoopin' workout in this position too. Who needs to pump iron? Jack, yes: Jill, no.

Side Swipin'

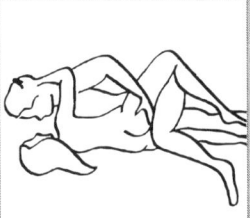

Jack and Jill are both in favorable positions, as all three-torso concepts are favored. A high five swipe for the Side Swipin' position? Jack, yes; Jill, yes.

Crouching Mister, Hidden Dragon Lady

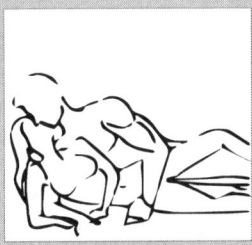

When morning breath takes away from morning romance, the Crouching Mister, Hidden Dragon Lady will help keep the lusty moment intact. This position is the alternative to Side Swipin'. He's crouching behind her; she's hidden under his cover. Jill will usually be the one to initiate the position. Is it safe to turn away from a Side Swipin' position? It sure is, for both partners! This position favors even more Torso Rhythm—so put the music on and let the dance party roll! With both facing in the same direction, Jack could make good use of his free hands. He could also help Jill get a little more feeling by pressing down on her leg. Just be careful with twisting torsos here because Twister is far from therapeutic. Jack and Jill get a lovin' yes for safety. Jack, yes; Jill, yes.

Surfboarding

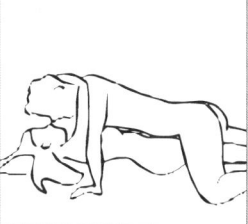

Jack is doing okay, floating and paddling his own way atop Jill toward his own splashing pinnacle. Jill, on the other hand, lies there as stiff as a Styrofoam plank. Styro girl is ready to crack anytime. Jill's torso has no room to rhythm, and unless she has the helping of Jack's five digits or a beach towel underneath the small of her back, the stiff surfer girl has no curves, either. If Jill wants more than her magic button rubbed, then she can tilt her pelvis up (which worsens Torso Curve) while Jack can jack himself into deeper waters. Jill, get out from under there! Summin' up this beach party: Jack is a yes, he's the hit of the party. Jill, on the other hand, should have stood him up instead. She's a no-no! If only Jack had been nice enough to place his lifejacket underneath her Torso Curve...he could have saved her! Jack, yes; Jill, hell no!

Fido's Pow Wow

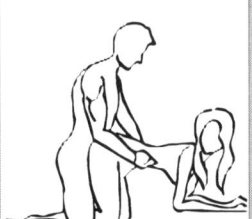

Wow, Jill is having the Pow Wow of her life. Jack, well, let's just say he's a lucky dog! Her Torso Threesome is maximized, safe to play all she wants. Jack is kneeling, which means gravity is a negative factor to consider if he wanders off too much from his lordosis. Bad doggy? Is he safe playing back there? Given that he has the freedom of Torso Curves, the freedom to contract his hoopers, and the freedom to move all he wants to the rhythm of Snoop Dogg, then gravity will have little to say about the safety of his moves. Go for it, as you both get a woofing yes! Jack, yes; Jill, yes.

Elevate-Her Wall-Bang-Her

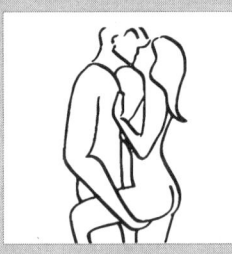

Who's sweatin' more here: you as examination taker, or Jack and Jill, passionately involved in advanced vertical "sexobics"? Assuming Jack is in good shape, good heart, good body proportions, good teeth and all, with no malignant "beer-belly-blastoma" that needs excision, then he's doing fine. The trick is for him to be able to keep with the low squatting position, maximize Torso Hoop, and go with Torso Rhythm and Curve until either the elevator starts moving again, or until they've both reached their top to yet another Penthouse letter. The trick with Jill is to use all of her Torso Hoop powers and single-powered thigh muscles to keep from toppling over to the floor, pulling Jack down with her and breaking Little Jack in half. Although very limited, Torsos Curve and Rhythm are not impossibilities, as long as she is self-powered (as opposed to having Jack hold her up at all times). Let the Elevate-Her Wall-Bang-Her be a new sport in the next Olympiad. Jack and Jill both get a high performance yes, and a gold medal to hang on their bedpost when they get home. Jack, yes; Jill, yes.

Heimlich Man Over

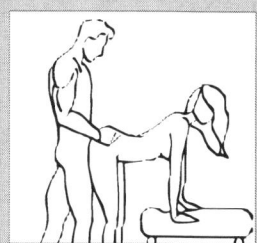 Jill is supporting herself with the chair, which helps eliminate the negative gravity pull on her low back as she leans over. All three torsos are safe at play, which means she really wasn't choking on anything after all. Jack's squat-hold is a mono-metric and very static position that re-

quires a hefty amount of low back hooper and thigh muscle strength. Since Mr. Heimlich's hands are busy helping Jill with her pleasures, he is compromising the safety of his low back hoopers. How long can he last? As he gets tired, his Torsos Curve and Rhythm will get low, shallow, and slow, which means he's going to be next in line for a strained and choking back Heimlich maneuver. If he had only used the armchair to hold himself, he'd be in the same boat as Jill, safe. Final answer? Jill will survive, and Jack will eventually collapse on top of Jill. Jill says: "Yes, yes!" and Jack says "Oh no! Down I go!"

Top of the Whirl

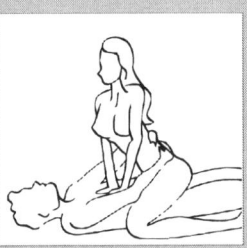

Jack is just lying there, not able to move very much. His Torso Curve and Torso Rhythm are minimal but still there if he concentrates and makes the effort. His job is to make sure he stays positioned well for Jill. Since their session is going to last longer than Stairway to Heaven, then Jack better use those hoopers and move along to the rhythm of Jill's humming. Jill is supporting herself on Jack. She's at the top of her world. It's all about her and she's got a go-ahead to climb right to the top of her inner world. Jack gets a marginal passing yes, while Jill gets a big yes right to her max!

Grenade Dive

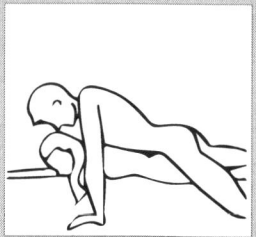

Jack is lying face down with as much Torso Curve and Rhythm as he wishes. He doesn't need much Torso Hoop strength in this position, unless he wanted to have a little workout at the same time he's shelling Jill. Jill may be protected from the grenade, but will she be shell shocked from having Jack's weight on top of her like that? If she had a pillow underneath her pelvis, her ride would be less bumpy because she would be able to keep her lumbar curve and rhythm. But she doesn't, and her safety is therefore compromised. Her rhythm is minimal because too much of it would make it difficult for Jack to keep his aim on Jill, let alone having to lift Jack with her tush in the air, a move called pelvic extension thrusts (But imagine the hoopin' low back workout she'd get!). So who survived the grenade blast? Jill gets a no and a Purple Heart medallion, while Jack gets a yes.

Hunk Her Down and Hunker Down

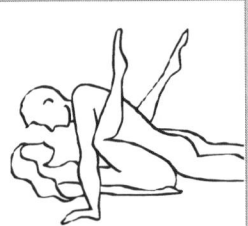

Jill is in serious trouble. After her hunk is done with the "hunking," she may decide to never hunker down again. Although this position favors Jill's stimulation as Jack lands himself perfectly onto her launch pad during every in and out, she should still forfeit the Hunker Down pose. Jill should just say no and leg press Jack right off her. Jack again has freedom of Torso Curve and Rhythm, with quite a bit of Torso Hoop action. Jill is doing all the pressing and Jack is the one getting a good workout. Jill should just say no, while Jack gets a pressing yes!

Lap Whacking

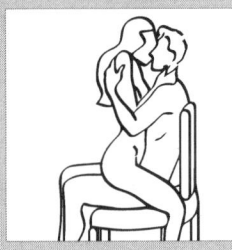

Jill is in the driver's seat this time. The only problem for Jill is, unless she's Xena's cousin, she's probably going on a very short driving trip. This thigh buster is very likely short lived because it's a grueling workout pose for Jill. This buster is also a step improved from Suzanne Somers' Thigh

Buster because it comes with fleshy accessories already assembled when delivered. The original Thigh Buster just doesn't sport anything but polyethylene and rubber accessories. Jill's got a lot of Torso Hoop action in this one, with quite a bit of Torso Curve and Rhythm control. Jack, on the other hand, may need to check himself into E.R. to get the splinters out of his ass. No matter how exciting the moment was, whicker pucks just aren't cool. Jack is stuck in a curveless torso position, with as much rhythm as the Pope's swing to the sounds of "Voulez Vous Coucher Avec Moi Ce Soir?" He also better have a good gut on him if he wants to make it out of the chair after Jill is done with her meat-patty whacking. What's the final judgment on the Lap Whacking? Jack gets a martyring no-no, and Jill sacrifices Jack's back for a satisfying yes!

Jack Hammer Hams Her

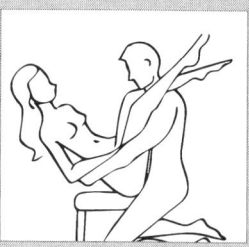 This one's for the most serious of lovemakers. Jack is in good shape here. His kneeling 'position actively involves all three-torso concepts. If more is said, it will just reflect further involvement of three other concepts I don't want to get into: envy, envy, and envy. So he gets a yes, yes, and yes. Jill, on

the other hand, is victimized by Jack's self-gratifying Sumo strapping hold. Give up, Jill? You should, because you have no way of even budging an inch to relieve the itch, strapped down not only with immobility but locked up in the worse alordosis pose. Jill gets a no go, and Jack gets a yes fest!

Rock-A-My-Baby-On-His-Tree-Stub

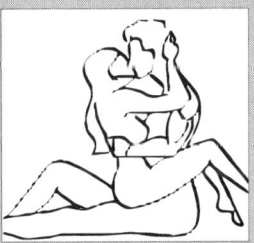

Other than a possible worst case of carpel tunnel syndrome, Jill gets a little yes. If she's very active, she will be capable of leaning back enough to create not only bobbing motion but also pelvic rhythm and curve with a good hoopin' workout. If she held the upright position, it would be more than her carpel tunnel she would be complaining about. Jack is leaning back, which helps relieve a bit of gravity-induced disc pressure. Jill is not exactly sitting on top of him, so he has some freedom of movement, as long as his little bonehead can take all the bending down. Jack, too, gets a little yes for this position, assuming he has the common sense to do what he's supposed to do to protect his back from breaking before her wrists do. If he wants to look extra good during his rock-a-my-baby moves, he'll also tighten up and work on his hoopers. Jack gets a teeny-weeny rockin' yes, and Jill gets a little-bitty bobbing yes, too.

Sling Shot Stir Ups

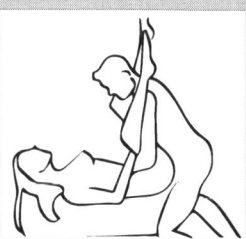

Jill is flat on her back, which quickly gets rid of all gravity effects on her flattened spine. Since her pelvis needs to be up for a proper glove fit, curves are sacrificed for stimulation and fitting fashions. Rhythm is kept to a minimum and Torso Hoop comes into play in a major big way if she's forced to hold things up herself. Two out of three ain't bad, and so, Jill gets a petite yes and a Grand Mal seizuring "Ohhhhh." Jack is leaning forward, which takes pressure off his low back as long as he leans onto Jill or the car hood, whichever is hotter. He's in control of his movements, which means there is plenty of Torso Curve and Rhythm. If he's smart, he will use his hoopers to help prevent tummy fumbling onto Jill's lower half. What's the answer for Jack? Yes Jack, of course you can safely play with the slingshot, just be careful where you point that thing. Jill, you can play slingshot with Jack too, but don't stay up too long!

TALLYING UP YOUR SEX SCORES

Minus Thirty to Plus Ten

Did you even read one page on the concepts of spinal safety? Consider yourself a student on probation with "not trustworthy to play with" noted in your transcript records. You are definitely not a safe one to play with. If you claim to be a more hands-on type of learner, I suggest you get your hands on yourself first and brush up on your masterlumbation sexercise techniques.

Eleven to Seventeen

So close, but still no cigar! There will be no smoking in your bed tonight. You still need to review the concepts of The Terrific Torso Threesome in order to be considered safe to play with. Don't give up!

Eighteen to Thirty

Congratulations! You know about Torso Curve, Rhythm, and Hoop, which means you understand the powers of the Sextitution in healing low back pain. You are a board-certified sexician. You are ready to take on a suffering patient. You can also be trusted to take on the wildest of sexual encounters while in the safety of your own, or your partner's Torso Curve, Rhythm and Hoop. Hoopla!

13

LOVE HURTS

When love poems turn to songs of despair, you know that Puffy is in pain. The inflammopath is hot. And when the inflammopath is hot...love hurts! The Sexy Back program is designed to help those burdened with chronic back pain—that's chronic, as in more than three months with little hope of it going away by itself. What's the difference between acute and chronic? You may look at acute as a passing storm, and chronic as the calm after. But there's also a price attached to acute when compared to chronic. The biggest difference between acute and chronic is about twelve hundred dollars when comparing the price of the "acute" emergency flight ticket on your way to New York from L.A., as opposed to the cost of a "chronic" well-planned-ahead reservation. Acute will always whip-slash your credit card. When consumed with tears on your pillow from the royal pain in your "Homo spinus," with little Homo erectus left to hold you up by the end of the day, you know you're acute. The consumed "inflammopathic" sufferer sucking on ice cubes to ease the spinal fever needs to know how to get by with a little lovin' until the beast within is calmed.

Bad enough to have to live by the infamous "love is blind" cliché, but when blinded love also becomes paralyzing from a sudden back panic attack, you know your love life is doomed. Your only escape is to know how to perform CPR on your own back until the beast leaves and your back pulse starts beating once again. Beauty from your front—beast from the back; you should learn how to keep your love life alive until the savage beast is soothed. The Sexy Back program is designed to fix The Guilty Triad and to give you the best excuse in the world to keep with the program. ("Again, I beg you, honey; Dr. Rice says you need to help me with this problem!") The Guilty Triad, if you remember, are the three factors related to the changing of our times that create—or will create—our modernized back problems. And with the triad comes differing degrees of pathologies, as described in the "Determinator" section of the book. With all of these dysfunctions may come acute episodic presentations that will turn you into a spontaneous 24/7 mess, with an unpredictable recovery plan. "Excuse me, miss, can you tell me when the plane to Pain Free Island will be landing?" "I'm sorry, sir, but we just don't know how much longer we will be circling the airport. Would you like a pillow?" Just get him a stiff drink for his spine!

Chronic, or sub-acute, pain means the pain has been there long enough to find "the beast" tolerable, but still irritable. It is during this time that you can participate in the In Vitro practicum and In Vivo practical parts of the Sexy Back program. When people start referring to you as "the global whiner" from all the acute debilitating back stabbing pains, you know you're not quite ready for the In Vitro and In Vivo programs.

LES MISÉRABLES

When you can't hide the grimace anymore, you have to learn to work your way around the facial uglies in order to get a bit of sexual endorphin release. Getting an auto-morphine fix will help ease the intensity of your back pain. Sexual positions exist that minimize spinal pressures while keeping with the rhythm of a passionate moment.

ARCHER OR TUCKER: THE PRINCIPLE OF THE CONTRAIREUR

In between all the "happy pill" digestion, served upon your very first lamenting cry for medical help, you will need to do more for yourself.

First, if extending (bending backwards, like you're doing the Demi on stage at Striptease) hurts more than leaning forward, then you will focus your acute pain relief moves on the Mean Pussycat pose (as often as you wish). If you do the Mean Pussycat pose lying on your back, it looks like you're pulling your knees to your chest—also an acceptable position! Getting relief from the Mean Pussycat pose makes you an "archer"—meaning your regular attitudinal pose is that of an overly exposed torso curve, which will cause irritation of your apophyseal joints (star points 3 and 5, articulating with the same numbers on the star above and below it).

If flexing (bending forward, like you're doing the Demi on stage at Striptease) hurts more than leaning backwards, then you will do multiples of the first sexercise for pain relief, the Push-up and Go Up, with no Mean Pussycat pose if you don't think you can get there. Getting relief from the push-up and Go Up moves makes you a "tucker," meaning that, like most out there, you keep your back in a flexed, alordotic position during most of your sitting time. This will irritate your vertebral discs, which will in turn express themselves in all kinds of wonderful ways.

The archer and tucker concept is called "The Principle of the Contraireur." It means that if you show tendencies toward being an archer type, then you do the exact opposite and become a tucker for back pain relief. If you have tendencies toward being the tucker type, then you do the opposite and become an archer for back pain relief when things get hot back there!

So you do the testing, you do the math, and you do your own therapy. Do these exercises on the hour for as long as you have sharp back pain shooting down and dragging you down. Besides, what else are you going to do after your doc cuts you off the drug fest orgy? "But doc, I'm still a cast member of 'Les 'Spinales' Misérables!'" Doc, where are you going? Isn't there a protective under-spray you can apply on a back like mine? Can't you just defuse this bomb inside my back? Don't you have a cure, doc? Come on, doc! You took an oath! I have questions. I have needs! Don't leave without giving me any drugs! Doc?" Sorry, but even Eminem's blue, yellow, and purple pills will take their toll after a while.

FEEL GOOD STRATEGIES

Apart from the sexercises, you are probably very familiar with other "feel good" therapies available for acute back pain. You know, "make me feel good" therapies that accessorize the pill popping routines, like icing, Dr. Ho's massager, Dr. Ho's acupressure point machine, Dr. Ho's topical analgesics, Epsom-salt baths, a bath with Dr. Ho, Dr. Ho's muscle stimulators, Dr. Ho's de-stress belt, etc… (Thank You, Dr. Ho!) And at your local pharmacy, there's more where these suggestions came from. That's what's become of pharmacies today. Their services are now more diversified than ever. More than a script drop-off and pick-up center, they have come out of their pharmaceutical cold storage closets and openly have helpful drug and therapeutic product talks with their clients. Take advantage!

The theme of Sexy Back stays in the bedroom, Thank You! Only climbing, grinding, pumping, nose-diving mean, and pussycats in these paragraphs. What is the best pain reliever of all times? The ones that come from within! It's the morphine-like chemical our brains secrete at the peak of our passion. How, then, can you lay yourself down, sustaining a lovemaking position long enough to open heaven's gates to endorphin land? Referring to the positions outlined in the previous section, "Examining All Options," let Jack (as in inadequate Jack) and Jill show how to get you some pain killing opiate release using a little lovin' when your back is more impotent than a marinated squid.

When Jack is in lamenting pain and all Jill wants is to play the game, there are three choices to pick from:

CHOICE A FOR WHEN JACK ACHES!

The Sling Shot Stir Ups is one position that favors Jack. Kneeling in front of Jill allows him three comforts. to keep with the lordosis, not putting any movement resistance against his rhythm, and if he's got the ab-power, then he can tighten up for greater protection. One important factor that helps keep the third wheel out of your bed (the angry Mr. Lumbar Jack!) is the availability to support himself with his arms using the sofa. Jill's legs are well strapped so he has little to do to keep her in her place. Thanks, Jill! And if Jack gets tired of playing with the sling shot, he can always "ham her with his hammer," the equivalent of the sling shot move.

CHOICE B FOR WHEN JACK ACHES!

Fido's Pow Wow: Choice B for when Jack's back stings like a bee! Wow, who would have guessed this position favored back pain! In case of an emergency, don't break back, just flip Jill over and calmly work your way toward the exit signs. Jill is well supported in this position, so Jack can concentrate on just his bracing needs, using her tush as a whacking cane.

CHOICE C FOR WHEN JACK ACHES!

Top of the Whirl: Choice C for when Jack's back is twingy and achy!

If Jack was debilitated to the point where, if it weren't for all the screaming, you'd think he was in a coma, then the position that favors absolute passivity is Top of the Whirl. Jack really should remember to place something in his Torso Curve area to maintain a lordosis during the whirling.

CHOICE A FOR WHEN JILL ACHES!

When Jill is wickedly acute, there are two faves to pick from:

Top of the Whirl: Choice One when Jill's the miserable one! Top of the Whirl is best because she is in absolute control to shake, rattle, and move without placing a lot of limits on the schmooze. She will be able to support herself well in this position, which helps reduce the workload on her lumbar erectors, keeping the disc pressure to a minimum.

CHOICE B FOR WHEN JILL ACHES!

Grenade Diving and Surfboarding: Choice Two when Jill can't be bothered to even lift a finger, let alone two legs.

If she's the one who looks like her back is in a coma, then she's better off lying on her stomach, preferably on the floor for a firm, less bouncy ride. In this position, Torso Curve is maxed out, which favors Jill big time, especially if she's on Sparky's team (sciatic irritations, for example). If her facets are the main source of discomfort (where bending backwards is way more difficult than forward), then all she has to do is place a few pillows underneath her pelvis or turn over, place a pillow in her

Torso Curve area, and play the role of Styro girl in the love story called Surfboarding. Don't worry, Jill, Jack promises two things that will make you happier: he will not put all of his weight on top of you and he will wake you up in time for "True Blood"!

THE BEST CHOICE FOR WHEN JACK & JILL ACHE!

When both Jack and Jill want to commit spinal suicide, there is still hope for keeping their union minimally gloomy. When both parties are occupied by hell-raising lumbars with a prescription of blue, yellow, and purple pills strong enough to kill an entire metal band, then only one position is favored if both suffering parties are to be pleased. To avoid the worst of he-howlings and she-shrieks, position choice is limited to Crouching Mister, Hidden Dragon Lady. In this position, you have two lamenting faces staring in the same direction like they're forced to watch C-Span. They who crouch together will painlessly stick together forever, or at least until the crouching mister and hidden dragon lady have climbed to the top of their mountain peaks.

If you really can't move at all, counting on your partner having to do all the driving, and not counting on ever getting a reservation on the next space shuttle launch to no-gravity delight, then here is the next best thing: lie on your back with a pillow underneath your knees (you figure it out) and a bit of packing in the Torso Curve area. Unless the other torso has a preference, legs spread or not won't make a difference.

One important message to keep in mind is that trauma, pain, and stress equally lessen the purity and concentration of sex hormones in both men and women. When sex "mones" are down, you can bet that sex moans are down as well! Libidos naturally go down when affected by these factors. This is caused by a reduction of male testosterone or female progesterone. No matter who's sitting on your lap, if you don't have the "mones" flowing through your veins, your brain is just not going to be in the game! Sometimes, "back-out" goes hand-in-hand with "time-out"!

SEX AND THE (NOT SO) SINGLE SPINE POP QUIZ

So what did you get out of this book? If you can answer yes to any of the following questions, I will be happy. If you can answer yes to all, I will be thrilled.

- Do you realize that you deserve to live a pain-free life?
- Do you understand that you have to get off your butt to help your back to heal?
- Did you learn four exercises to help you end your back pain?
- Do you understand that you deserve to have and enjoy sex?
- Do you know and understand that sex will help you reduce pain and heal your back?

Read this book over and over again until the answer to all is: YES!

14

WAS IT AS GOOD FOR
YOU AS IT WAS FOR ME?

I get up at 5:41 a.m.. I do it out of respect for the other
Five-Forty-Oners waiting for me at the end of my first 5K,
and I do it for me. Getting up this morning was easier than
most days but when I met a dozen other Five-Forty-Oners
outside the front gates of dumbbell land, I discovered the
best excuse in the world not to work out: Not my fault, the
gym never opened!

Content to head back to the unmade king size I left
behind at 5:41, I faced south, then east, and then realized
I really was already where I needed to be. Not lying in my
king size prize, but facing my very own sunrise. And at
6:02 you can safely call it your own.

At this time of the morning she's friendly, romantic, and has a lot of free time to share a petit café et croissant with you. At that early hour, when I stared into the friendly pink hue above me, it perfectly tinted my sunglasses rose.

You do it too.

You hold your gaze, a daring stare that allows her enough time to have its effect on you: scorching stress, melting madness, drying out despair, and roasting reality. She molds what matters and cooks what counts.

During the day we seek protection from her powers. Over the years, fear and wit have forced us into a new Darwinian era, changing from sun worshippers to sunscreen lovers. Anything less than Factor 30 sunscreen and 100% UV Protection glasses are considered completely careless, utterly irresponsible and downright self-abusive. We fear her and we love her.

But this morning, she changes face and becomes all friendly again—all mine to play with! Playful and happy, like the beaming energy of a child that stays with you long after he's left looking for Spiderman adventures. She is your morning breakfast spirit that will leave you a long-lasting happy, childlike spirit for the rest of your day.

"Nutri-men" say that your early morning feeding is the most important meal of the day. But at that time in the morning, looking her right in the eye, she's telling you something bigger than what could ever fill the bowls of your innermost self-dialogue. Are you listening to what she's telling you? This is what I hear her say: "It's not that complicated anymore. Hold on to today; nothing is that complicated. Hold off on tomorrow, as it is not with us today!"

Got it! The galaxy queen has spoken!

The list of things we are to love is not as long as we think it is. When it's just you and her, fallen egos and cracked competitiveness need not be repaired. You can ignore the trying impact of all those things burning away your childlike enthusiasm during your day. You can count on her feeding you all the essential awakenings that take the day's bellyaches away. At this time of the morning I love myself, I love being alive, I love my family and friends and the simplicity of life.

I am not daunted that I really am in a world so unaffected by my existence.

You should feel like this.

I wake up at 5:41. A Five-Forty-Oner can stare her in the face and take in her awakening punch. "Happy to be alive" offerings will last the whole day! She's the best hostess ever. Life is being served at 5:41. Get up, eat up, and digest, will ya?

I have had long discussions with my son Chris, about the beauty of our "selves." This son of mine knows about the "nothingness" that we really are on this satellite-decorated planet that is everyone's right to live on. Although we are part of the "everything under the sun," we are also nothing to anything that has real meaning.

Grim sounds from a future man.

I want to pass my fatherly native wisdom to my son: "The special thing that you think you are can only be so if you make others around you feel just as special. Passing it on is how you pack on meaning to being everything under the sun, son."

Become a Five-Forty-Oner. Let her stare you in the face long enough to wake a change in you. Let her burn away the unimportant and flare up the little you that you are, turning you into a "spiritual giver of special auras."

You have a right to live your life in hope. Without fear. Without pain.

Embrace this life. It is yours.

Written at 5:41 a.m.,

in her company,

over a petit déjeuner.

Dr. Michel Rice

TESTIMONIALS

DR ALEJANDRO ESPALDA | SWEDEN

"Sexy Back is a medical self-help book on chronic lower back pain. It is both educating and entertaining at the same time. Who knew this could be possible. Dr. Rice I guess!"

DR HO | TELEVISION SHOPPING NETWORK US & CANADA

"Dr. Rice is an expert on research and low back pain. This take on back pain is original and entertaining. People will enjoy it and learn a lot about their backs."

DRS ERIC AND DYAN DUPAYA | CHICAGO

"This approach to back pain is both academic and fun. When we teach doctors in training, we use the same techniques. It allows for long term memory anchoring. Patients will really enjoy the Sexy Back read and learn all the spinal essentials.

Yes patients will enjoy learning what there is to know about their backs all taught in a fun yet comprehensive way."

Rx

DR. MICHEL RICE
TORONTO ON
WWW.SEXYBACKDOCTOR.COM

PATIENT NAME: _____

DATE: _____

Rx Chronic Low Back Pain

Rx Get!

Dr Rice

SIGNATURE

Rx

DR. MICHEL RICE
TORONTO ON
WWW.SEXYBACKDOCTOR.COM

PATIENT NAME: _____

DATE: _____

Rx Chronic Low Back Pain

ATT:
Holder of this prescription
is authorized to help
you with your back pain

Dr Rice

SIGNATURE